Working in Health Care
WHAT YOU NEED TO KNOW TO SUCCEED

Working in Health Care

WHAT YOU NEED TO KNOW TO SUCCEED

Michael W. Drafke, EdD
Professor, College of DuPage
Glen Ellyn, Illinois

F. A. Davis Company • Philadelphia

F. A. Davis Company
1915 Arch Street
Philadelphia, PA 19103
www.fadavis.com

Printed in the United States of America

Last digit indicates print number: 10 9 8 7 6 5 4

Acquisitions Editor: Margaret Biblis
Developmental Editor: Rose G. Foltz
Production Editor: Nwakaego Fletcher-Perry
Cover Designer: Louis Forgione

As new scientific information becomes available through basic and clinical research, recommended treatments and drug therapies undergo changes. The author(s) and publisher have done everything possible to make this book accurate, up to date, and in accord with accepted standards at the time of publication. The author(s), editors, and publisher are not responsible for errors or omissions or for consequences from application of the book, and make no warranty, expressed or implied, in regard to the contents of the book. Any practice described in this book should be applied by the reader in accordance with professional standards of care used in regard to the unique circumstances that may apply in each situation. The reader is advised always to check product information (package inserts) for changes and new information regarding dose and contraindications before administering any drug. Caution is especially urged when using new or infrequently ordered drugs.

Library of Congress Cataloging-in-Publication Data

Drafke, Michael, W.
    Working in health care : what you need to know to succeed / Michael W. Drafke.—[2nd ed.].
        p. cm.
    Includes index.

    1. Allied health personnel—Practice. I. Title
R729 .D73 2002
610.69′53—dc21

                                                    2001047903

ISBN 13: 978-0-8036-0965-5
    ISBN 10: 0-8036-0965-5

Dedicated to my three sons, Adam, Erik, and Alex;
my wife, Kathleen; my father and mother,
Raymond and Jeanette; and the rest of my family.

Preface

The idea for this book came from my observation that—other than the technical skills needed to perform a certain job—few workers understand much about working. Few workers understand how management works, what the roles of a manager and a worker are, or what is involved in organizational behavior. Many people do not know how to work effectively with their coworkers. As the working world, especially health care, began to change, the need for an organized introduction to working seemed necessary.

The first action I took was to create a course for the College of DuPage Radiography Program to address the topics that appear in this book. When I first presented the course to the program's advisory committee, someone asked, "Don't people learn these things on the job or during clinical?" My answer was that a few do, but most do not. This seemed too important a topic to leave to chance or to "learning by accident." Over the years, many students enrolled in this new course remarked that topics they had never thought about or that they never understood were covered and explained. The response to this class led to my writing this book.

I have two main goals in writing this book. First, I want to produce a book for health-care professionals that explains the nontechnical aspects of working in health care. I want health-care workers to understand how to work with others and with management: I want people to understand some of the reasons they do things and some of the reasons others do things. (As a joke, my working title for the book was "How to Work With Others Without Wanting to Strangle Them.") My aim is to improve coworker relations and manager-managee relations. I had to invent the term "managee" to describe someone who has a manager; the management terms—worker, subordinate, and so on—were all too negative.

My second main goal is to get people to read it. If people do not read the book, then accomplishing the first goal is meaningless. I decided to write directly to the reader in a simple, even casual, style. I believe the book will benefit more people if it is less dry and more readable. That said, let me assure everyone—this book and the material in it are quite serious.

So, to all readers, study this book, learn its lessons, and apply those lessons. Your job satisfaction and more may be at stake. Enjoy your work and be the best "managee" you can be.

Michael Drafke, EdD

Acknowledgments

First, I must thank my wife, Kathleen. I am not sure if it is harder to write a book, or to live with someone who is writing a book. I also thank the following reviewers of the first edition for their suggestions.

Karen Jacobs, MS, OTR/L
Adjunct Clinical Professor
Department of Occupational Therapy
Boston University
Boston, Massachusetts

Terrie Nolinske, MA, OTR/L, CO
Assistant Professor
Department of Occupational Therapy
St. Luke's Medical Center
Chicago, Illinois

Elizabeth M. Kanny, MA, OTR/L
Lecturer and Head
Department of Occupational Therapy
University of Washington
Seattle, Washington

Edith Carter Fenton, MS, OTR/L
Coordinator
Department of Occupational Therapy Assisting
Becker Junior College
Worcester, Massachusetts

Lynn Lippert, MS, PT
Chair of Physical Therapy Program
Mt. Hood Community College
Gresham, Oregon

Leonard Elbaum, PT, MM
Professor
Department of Physical Therapy
Florida International University
Miami, Florida

Thomas Schmitz, PhD, PT
Assistant Professor
Long Island University
Brooklyn, New York

Anna Parkman, MBA, RRT
Associate Professor and Program Coordinator
Respiratory Therapy Program
University of Charleston
Charleston, West Virginia

Peggy Burrows, MS, RT(R)
Clinical Instructor
Department of Radiologic Technology
Genessee Hospital
Rochester, New York

Mary Jane Clarke, MS, RT(R)
Director of Radiography Program
Quinnipiac College
Hamden, Connecticut

Gay Golden, MEd, RT
Department of Medical Imaging
University of Alabama, Health Related Professions
Birmingham, Alabama

Steven Dowd, MA, RT(R)
Program Director
Department of Radiologic Technology
University of Alabama
Birmingham, Alabama

Patricia J. Duffy, MPS, RT(R)
Assistant Director/Clinical Coordinator
Department of Radiologic Technology
State University of New York
Syracuse, New York

Last, but not least, I thank the entire staff at F. A. Davis Company, especially Lynn Borders Caldwell and Jean-François Vilain, for their help with the first edition, and Margaret Biblis and Rose Foltz for their help with the second edition. Few realize how many people (production, editorial, secretarial, marketing, and so on) are vital to the creation of a book.

Contents

1 ○ Why People Work

Objectives

On completion of this chapter, the reader will be able to:

☐ Define professional employee.

☐ Define work.

☐ Differentiate between work and play.

☐ Identify the reasons why people work.

☐ Explain employer theories of why people work.

On first inspection this may seem to be an odd chapter. After all, we all know why we work, and we know the difference between when we are working and when we are playing. Or do we? Explaining the difference between work and play is not so easy. The same is true when we examine the reasons why people work. Everyone knows that people work for money. At least that is what most people say if you ask them. However, money is not the only reason why people work. Understanding why people work is the first step to becoming a professional employee.

This book is devoted to helping you become a professional employee. A professional employee is not simply someone who is paid to work. Nor is it someone who belongs to a "profession." A professional employee is someone who is educated about what it means to work and to be a worker.

Many people "go to work," but few understand the myriad forces that affect work and the worker. A professional employee does. A professional employee knows the difference between a good working environment and a poor one—*and can explain the difference.* A professional employee understands the role of the worker and the role of management. A professional employee knows what contributes to his or her job satisfaction, knows how to cope with change, and understands motivation,

communication, and stress factors. Possibly most important of all, a professional employee knows how to work with others and how to be an asset to his or her employer.

These and other important topics are covered in this book. Learning the material presented here should help you derive greater benefit from and achieve more throughout your career. There is another reason, however, to learn the material in this book—the tendency now and for the foreseeable future is for "professional employees" to be more highly valued by employers. With trends toward empowerment and self-management, emphasis on customer service and total quality control, and reductions in the number of middle managers, employers are relying more and more on each employee to know many more aspects of how organizations function. While investigating these and other topics, we must also examine why people choose to work and have a career at all.

What Is Work?

Before answering this question, please complete Building Comprehension Exercise 1–1.

BUILDING COMPREHENSION EXERCISE 1–1

Differentiating Work and Play

Write what you believe are the differences between work and play.

Work is: _____

_____

_____

Play is: _____

_____

_____

Check your ideas with the following text.

End of exercise. Text continues on following page.

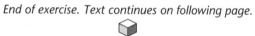

Everyone knows when he or she is working or, alternately, playing. However, when asked to explain the difference between work and play, most people have a difficult time of it.

Some say they know they're working because they're being paid money for their efforts. However, payment cannot be used as a criterion to distinguish work from play because it would then follow that cleaning one's own house, changing the oil in one's car, or doing one's laundry would be classified as play.

Maybe the difference between work and play is that working means doing something that you do not like. However, applying this standard is not always sufficient to differentiate work from play. In fact, although it is socially acceptable for people to dislike their jobs, in reality, most people like the work they do, or at least significant aspects of it.[1] Therefore, because many people enjoy their work, liking or disliking a task is not a reliable means of differentiating work and play activities. Nor can we examine a task by itself to find the difference. Playing sports may be recreation to you, but it is work to a professional athlete.

To find the difference between work and play, we must examine three factors *together:*

1. The *purpose* of the activity
2. The *attitude* of the person engaged in the activity
3. The *rewards* received from performing the activity

The difference, then, is in *you* and in *your reason* for doing an activity.[2]

Work is purposeful activity.[3] On the other hand, play does not need a purpose. Work accomplishes something. Something is created, changed, or destroyed. Work has an outcome.

But, the preceding standard by itself is still not a sufficient definition because play sometimes leads to an outcome too. For example, landscaping a backyard is play to some people, and it has an outcome. However, to a professional landscaper it is work. Thus, for an activity to be classified as work, the *attitude* of the person engaged in it must be that the activity is, indeed, work.

When the same purposeful activity can be viewed as work by some and play by others, we must also look at the type of reward—external or internal—a person receives to help us differentiate between the two. Work earns *external* reward; that is, those rewards received from other people. The most common external reward is money, although praise, recognition, status, and a promotion are also external rewards. In contrast, the rewards for play are *internal*. Internal rewards are derived inside the person from performing the activity. Examples of internal rewards are enjoyment, satisfying one's curiosity, and meeting one's altruistic goals.

Why People Work

Being able to differentiate between work and play does not explain why people work. Ask most people why they work and they say "For money." After all, it seems to be the most obvious answer. But people do not want money alone. First of all, what people really want are all the things that money can buy. Money is an accepted form of payment because it facilitates the transaction of goods. It enables us to exchange our labor for the things we need and want. It is much easier to trade $20 for some gasoline than it is to try to exchange a respiratory therapy treatment for some premium unleaded. It should be noted that there are a few people for whom money is merely a way of keeping score. These people have and make vast quantities of money. For them, money's everyday utility has been lost; it just tells them how well or how poorly they are doing that day. For most of us, though, money is really just one reason for working and—as we shall see in Chapter 11, Job Satisfaction— a frequently misunderstood one at that.

A number of explanations have been proposed to answer the question of why people work. One anonymous explanation is that people work because work is the best way anyone has yet found to fill a large space of time. There is certainly some validity to this as anyone who has been unemployed (completely without work, school, child-rearing, and so on) can tell you. Many people will say that having absolutely nothing to do loses its allure after 2 to 3 weeks. After this, people may become listless, unmotivated, and depressed. Without work there is no reason to go to bed at any particular time because there is no need to get up the next morning at any particular time. Soon procrastination becomes the rule. After all, there is plenty of time, so why do today what can be put off until tomorrow? Being without work means having to watch your money, and you soon discover that walking to the library is one of the few things that you can do for free. When unemployed, we quickly find we get more from work than simply being able to pay the bills.

What then are the reasons for working? In virtually all societies there are strong moral reasons for work. The moral reasons were first stated by Martin Luther in the 1500s.[4] Essentially, reasons for work were considered by Luther and his followers in a

BUILDING COMPREHENSION EXERCISE 1–2

Why Do You Work?

Rank the following reasons why you work, with 1 being the most important reason. Use the spaces in the Present Rank *column. Write in additional reasons if you need to.*

Present Rank   **Future Rank**

_____   1. To help others   _____

_____   2. To set your own goals   _____

_____   3. To be promoted   _____

_____   4. For an annual raise   _____

_____   5. For benefits   _____

_____   6. To obtain power   _____

_____   7. For a status job title   _____

_____   8. To learn (on the job)   _____

_____   9. For a feeling of achievement   _____

_____   10. To get money (salary)   _____

_____   11. For recognition   _____

_____   12. To receive feedback   _____

_____   13. For a feeling of success   _____

_____   14. To have responsibility   _____

_____   15. To perform interesting work   _____

_____   16. _____   _____

_____   17. _____   _____

_____   18. _____   _____

Exercise continues on following page 🎲🎲🎲

Money (item 10) was probably your number 1 reason for working (or was very close to being number 1). How is it possible to make this prediction without knowing you personally? Write your answer here and compare it to the answer below.*

_____

_____

*You may have said that everyone wants money, which is only partially true, as will be seen in the following section. You may have said that you need money to live, which is true, but is that the most important reason for working? You may have ranked money high because, if you are a student, you probably do not have much money right now.

Now, imagine yourself 10 or 15 years from now, earning enough money to live in your own home, own a respectable car, and have a reasonable number of possessions. Rank the reasons you think will be important to you then using the Future Rank column. How have your answers changed from your present rankings?

End of exercise. Text continues on following page.

religious, moral context. This set of beliefs came to be known as the "Protestant work ethic." Today the spiritual reasons are less prominent,[5] having been replaced by working mainly to attain the "American Dream."[6] In other words, people today work to attain their goals rather than to attain good standing in God's eyes. However, one holdover remains from the religious work ethic: It is still more socially acceptable to work than to be idle. This belief is held widely, creating a certain amount of peer pressure on people to work continuously.

Another theory concerning why people work was presented by Douglas McGregor.[7] He said that work is a person's natural state. To be alive means to be active. Some of that activity is play, and some is work. It is rather like saying "I am; therefore I work."

Max Weber[8] asked a question that is related to McGregor's theory. Weber wanted to know whether we lived to work or worked to live. A moralist might say that we live to work. A modern union member might say that we work to live.[9] It is possible that the answer is not important. The fact is that people work. Indeed, numerous studies have shown that people would continue to work even if they had the financial means not to work.[10] For whatever reason or reasons, the answer to the question of why people work is that work satisfies certain human needs.

What are these needs and which of them may be satisfied through work? One of the most widely accepted explanations of human needs was developed by Abraham Maslow.[11] Maslow identified categories of needs and arranged them in a hierarchy

(Fig. 1–1). The hierarchical arrangement means that the lower level needs must be met before a person even realizes that the next higher level need even exists. Maslow found five general needs: phys-0 iologic, safety, belonging, status and self-esteem, and self-actualization.

The physiologic needs are the most basic; they must be fulfilled before a person would even realize there are higher needs. The physiologic needs are those for the basics to maintain life—food, shelter, clothing, and water. Without these, we would not care about any of the other needs. For example, if you were stranded on an island without food, shelter, clothing, and water, you would not really care about whether you had a Timex watch or a $10,000 Rolex watch. (You might not even care whether you had a watch at all!)

Once their physiologic needs are met (or nearly so), people then realize the need for safety. This need is to feel physically safe and secure from threats and danger. To use the desert island metaphor, sitting high in a tree might ensure one's safety, but safety is not important if there is no food and one is in danger of starving to death.

Once physiologic and safety needs are met, the next needs you would become aware of are the belonging needs. These include the need to be with others and the need to have a mate. These two needs can be traded off with each other somewhat. People who have not yet found a mate may increase the number of friends and other social contacts they have. Once a mate is found, contact with friends may decrease. It is as if we each have our own level of need to be with others, and we can meet that need in one of two ways. We may meet our level all with friends, with our mate, or with a balance of friends and our mate.

The next level concerns status and self-esteem. It seems that once our need to be with others is met, we then feel the need to be better than they are! We each want a certain level of status within the group we see regularly, and we each need to reach a certain level of self-esteem to feel good about ourselves. Maslow felt that many people reach this level but do not progress to the last level—self-actualization.

Self-actualization is probably best explained by the United States Army slogan, "Be all that you can be." Self-actualization means that you push yourself to achieve the most that you can possibly achieve. This would include learning the most that you can, all of the time, and applying yourself to the best of your abilities, all of the time. This doesn't mean you never relax, but it does mean that you do not become comfortable with what you currently know and do the minimum to get by. Maslow was probably right— not many people are

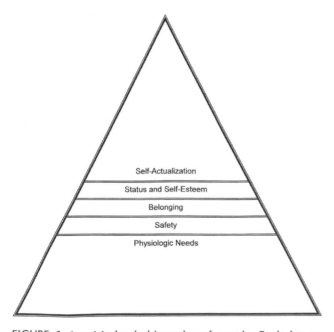

FIGURE 1–1 • Maslow's hierarchy of needs. Each lower-level need must be fulfilled (or nearly fulfilled) before people realize that there are higher needs. Once a need is fulfilled, it will no longer motivate anyone.

willing to push themselves to their limits and to expand those limits most of the time. Many people reach a certain level that they can live with, then grab the remote and hit the couch.

These are the five levels of Maslow's basic hierarchy of needs. He later revised his theory, saying that there are three other needs off to the side of the basic hierarchy that some people feel.[12] These are the needs for knowledge, comprehension, and aesthetics. Feeling the need for knowledge refers to the accumulation of facts. Maslow felt that certain people seemed more curious to know things. To this person, virtually every book in a bookstore or library looks interesting.

Comprehension was defined as the need to find the relationship among facts. For example, when a product like a sports car becomes more commercially available, it loses its appeal to some people. Some people might not care why this is so, whereas others would be quite curious to know why. (It's because the sports car has lost status by being widely available. Status is based on only a few people being able to have something; if everyone can have one, people with high-status needs often no longer desire it.)

The third additional factor Maslow mentioned is the need for aesthetics. This is the need for things to have a pleasing style or design. This would include the need to have a functional design, balance, or artistic design. Rectangular glass-covered office buildings, a delivery van, or a sweatsuit would not receive high ratings for being aesthetically pleasing from most people. A Frank Lloyd Wright building, a Lamborghini Diablo, or an Armani tuxedo probably would.

Theories of Work

Employers have also examined the question of why people work, and they seem to follow one of two theories. Some follow the first half of Weber's question: Do we live to work, or work to live? Others follow the second half.

Some bosses and institutions believe in the theory that people live to work (I work; therefore I am). In their view of the world, people are there to fulfill the company's need for workers.[13] They believe that work is the single most important thing in a person's life—and, it is way ahead of whatever is in second place. As their employee, you should be prepared to give 110 percent to the company. You should be prepared to come in early and stay late or take work home, as the job requires. You go home at night to rest up for the next day's work. You are expected to leave your private life outside the workplace, and nothing should interfere with your work hours. Some are just short of believing that because they employ you, they own you. Unfortunately, some of these organizations that expect total loyalty and devotion will not reciprocate. They readily lay employees off at the first sign of economic trouble. When it comes to work performance problems, this type of organization is more likely to have the attitude that you produce or you are fired. There is a tendency to let you work out your own problems. Often, their final view is, "if you don't like it here, leave."

At the opposite end of the spectrum are the employers who believe that work is only a part of life. They believe you have a life outside of work,[14] including, for example, a family, other interests, and other responsibilities. These are the employers that are more likely to have variable starting times for the workday. They are more likely to give employees personal time off or a "mental health day." They are more likely to offer employee assistance programs, and they realize that events in other parts of your life can affect your work temporarily. Some may take this one step further with the belief that anything that affects your work is your boss's concern. They believe they should intervene, whether you want them to or not. Some encourage single people to marry, believing that a married person is a more stable, mature worker with more energy to give to work (and the belonging needs are met, so the married person is one step closer to self-actualization). The overall attitude of concern for employees and respect for the impact the rest of their lives can have on their job performance can work quite well, but both managers and employees must remember that productivity still counts.

When interviewing an employer for a job, try to ascertain where the boss and the institution fall between these extremes, and determine whether or not you would be satisfied working in such a system.

Summary

This chapter introduces the basic concept of work, the reasons why people work, and work theories. Some of the theories of work can help identify the organization's philosophy toward employees so that you can match that philosophy with the kind under which you would like to work. This chapter is also part of the foundation for Chapters 4, 5, 6, and 8.

When thinking about the broad ideas presented here, you may discover what many people have already discovered; that is, they have a love-

 Building Comprehension Exercise begins on following page

Understanding Maslow's Hierarchy

For each of the levels of Maslow's Hierarchy, describe how well work fulfills your needs and how it does this. For how well work satisfies your needs, FS means work Fully Satisfies this need, MS means work Mostly Satisfies this need, SS means work Somewhat Satisfies this need, CAL means work Contributes A Little to satisfying this needs, and DS means work Doesn't Satisfy this need.

Self-Actualization Needs

How well work satisfies this need   FS   MS   SS   CAL   DS

Describe how work satisfies this need:

_____

_____

_____

_____

_____

Status and Self-Esteem Needs

How well work satisfies this need   FS   MS   SS   CAL   DS

Describe how work satisfies this need:

_____

_____

_____

_____

_____

Belonging Needs

How well work satisfies this need   FS   MS   SS   CAL   DS

Describe how work satisfies this need:

_____

_____

_____

Exercise continues on following page ❖ ❖ ❖

_____

_____

Safety Needs

How well work satisfies this need   FS   MS   SS   CAL   DS

Describe how work satisfies this need:

_____

_____

_____

_____

_____

Physiologic Needs

How well work satisfies this need   FS   MS   SS   CAL   DS

Describe how work satisfies this need:

_____

_____

_____

_____

_____

Now, describe how you _might_ fulfill those needs you rated SS, CAL, or DS from activities within work (like working toward a promotion) and from outside of work (like volunteering).

_____

_____

_____

_____

_____

Finally, circle those items that you feel you are most likely to use to fulfill your unmet needs. These items can be used as the basis for forming your personal goals.

End of exercise. Text continues on following page.

hate relationship with work.[15] It seems that work is difficult to live with and difficult to live without. However, contemplating why we do or do not work can lead to other questions that most people might prefer not to think about. If you consider why you work, then eventually you might consider not working. But if you don't work, what do you do? What is your reason for being here? What do you do with the knowledge you have accumulated? Why bother to learn anything new if you are not going to put your skills to use? Working may suddenly appear to be not so bad, even if you have work rather than a calling (which many people seem to be seeking).[16] So, it may be simpler to just work rather than to face the answers to the questions not working can present.

REFERENCES

1. Maccoby, M, and Terzi, K: What happened to the work ethic? In Hoffman, MW, and Wyly, T (eds): The Work Ethic in Business. Oelgeschlager, Gunn, and Hain, Cambridge, Mass., 1981, pp 31–32.
2. Smith, HC, and Wakely, JH: Psychology of Industrial Behavior, ed 3. McGraw-Hill, New York, 1972, p 38.
3. Ibid, p 37.
4. Cherrington, M: The Work Ethic: Working Values and Values That Work. AMACOM, New York, 1980, p 20.
5. Yankelovich, D: New Rules: Searching for Self Fulfillment in a World Turned Upside Down. Bantam Books, New York, 1982, p 7.
6. Ibid, p 8.
7. Smith, and Wakely, p 37.
8. Weber, M: The Theory of Social and Economic Organization. Henderson, AM, and Parsons, T (trans). Free Press, New York, 1947, p 329.
9. Tyler, Gus: The work ethic: A union view. In The Work Ethic: A Critical Analysis. Industrial Relations Research Association, Madison, Wisc., 1983, p 197.
10. Maccoby, and Terzi, p 34.
11. Maslow, AH: Motivation and Personality. Harper & Row, New York, 1954.
12. Maslow, AH: Motivation and Personality, ed 3. Harper & Row, New York, 1970.
13. O'Reilly, B: Is your company asking too much? Fortune, March 12, 1990, pp 38–46.
14. Levering, R, and Moskowitz, M: The 100 best companies to work for. Fortune, January 10, 2000, pp 82–110.
15. Maccoby, and Terzi, p 33.
16. Labich, K: Kissing Off Corporate America. Fortune, February 20, 1995, p 44.

2 ◦ The Work Environment

○ *Chapter Outline*

Objectives

On completion of this chapter, the reader will be able to:

☐ Define terms used to describe the work environment.
☐ Differentiate between the physical and mental work environments.
☐ Differentiate between factors within the physical work environment.
☐ Differentiate between factors within the mental work environment.
☐ Show how the physical work environment can affect a person.
☐ Show how the mental work environment can affect a person.
☐ Explain how an individual can affect his or her mental and physical work environments.

There are two aspects to the work environment, the physical and the mental. The *physical work environment* consists of the equipment and surroundings in which the employees must function. The *mental work environment* is the psychological atmosphere in which the employees must operate. Both of these affect the employee's work and satisfaction (Fig. 2–1).

The Physical Work Environment

Potential employees often overlook the physical work environment when applying for a job unless it is overwhelmingly good or bad. Usually they notice the environment only after being on the job for some time. Many times a poor physical work

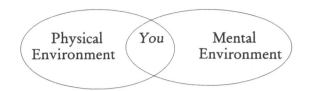

FIGURE 2–1 • Both the physical and mental environments affect you (the employee).

environment results in inefficiency, unnecessary fatigue, low morale, increased turnover and absenteeism, lost time, and low productivity.[1] It is important that management and employees recognize when a poor physical environment is the cause of these or other problems. Only when you have properly identified the problem can you correct it. Otherwise you may end up manipulating or complaining about the wrong factors, leaving the real problem unresolved. Resolving physical work environment problems benefits clients or patients and management, as well as workers.

You may also be dissatisfied with your job because of a poor physical environment. Knowing how the physical environment can affect people will allow you to identify the source of the dissatisfaction and address it. Otherwise, you might attribute the dissatisfaction to something that is not really the problem (the work, the boss, pay, coworkers). Proper identification of the source of a problem is the first step toward resolving it. The factors of the physical environment that affect people are:

- Temperature and humidity
- Ventilation
- Light
- Noise
- Location
- Space
- Layout
- Equipment
- Supplies
- Color and decor
- Comfort
- Security
- Social contacts

In a health-care environment, these factors must also be considered from the patient's point of view.

TEMPERATURE AND HUMIDITY

Temperature and humidity can be considered together in their effects on worker and patient comfort. For the tasks performed by most health-care

workers, the range for the maximum temperature is 77°F to 81°F.[2] Seated workers could tolerate a maximum temperature of about 86°F. Those performing heavier physical labor are usually more comfortable at a maximum temperature of 72°F. The minimum temperature for health workers should be about 65°F.[3] Temperatures below 50°F and above 86°F can have serious adverse effects on work—for example, fatigue, difficulty with fine motor skills, and decreased ability to concentrate. A comfortable range for humidity is 40 to 60 percent. For optimum comfort, humidity should decrease as temperature increases. Whereas most hospital workers are comfortable with these temperature and humidity ranges, many patients are not. Workers are constantly moving, generating their own heat. Patient movement is almost always restricted. It is also common for patients to be dressed lightly. Therefore, many patients are cold when the health workers are comfortable, or the workers are too warm when the patients are comfortable. One common solution is to keep the temperature closer to the worker levels and keep patients covered with blankets. Another option is to zone the patient and employee areas. When zoning is used, each area (the nurse's station, laboratory, employee lounges, and so on) has its own temperature controls, allowing more people to be comfortable more often.

VENTILATION

Ventilation is important in maintaining productivity, morale, and a healthy environment.[4] It is especially important in the closed and often windowless environs of today's architecture. Room air should be changed 4 to 10 times per hour.[5] The air should be changed so that it does not create a draft, and it should circulate often enough so that the room does not become stagnant. Adequate ventilation can help reduce the claustrophobia that some workers and patients experience.

Areas with strong odors require extra ventilation or deodorization, or both. The federal government requires posted warnings in work areas containing hazardous fumes, and, depending on the substances involved, Occupational Safety and Health Administration (OSHA) regulations may require that safety equipment be worn. Patients are often more sensitive to odors; therefore, cleanliness and liberal use of deodorants will make the environment more pleasant for everyone.

LIGHT

Adequate lighting for most work situations is near 10 footcandles, which is equal to the light emitted

BUILDING COMPREHENSION EXERCISE 2–1

Assessing the Physical Work Environment

Examine your current work environment. Which of these factors could be changed relatively easily? Which do you think should be changed? How would you change the factor?

Physical Work Environment Factors	Could Be changed	Should Be changed	How should this factor be changed?
Temperature			
Humidity			
Ventilation			
Light			
Noise			
Department location			
Space			
Layout			
Equipment			
Supplies			
Color			
Decor			
Your comfort			
Security			
Social contacts			

End of exercise. Text continues on following page.

by a 40-watt light bulb that is 2 ft away.[6] This does vary significantly, with typical surgical procedures requiring over 500 footcandles of light.[7] Increasing amounts of light can contribute to increasing productivity. For example, Tinker,[8] in 1939, found that when lighting was increased from 2.4 to 11 footcandles, there was a 15 percent increase in productivity. Lighting does follow the law of diminishing returns, however. Increasing the amount of light produces smaller and smaller increases in benefits.[9]

Contrast and ambient-to-work lighting should also be considered when examining lighting.[10] When the contrast between objects is high, less illumination is required. For example, greater accuracy with less lighting is achieved when reading black numbers on a white dial compared with gray numbers on a white dial. Accuracy is also greatest when the ratio of ambient (room) lighting to lighting on the work object is 1 to 1. It is easier to read equipment or perform work when the illumination of the object is equal to room light. Also, green light produces less fatigue than other colors.[11]

Much more could be done with lighting by keeping the patient and family comfort in mind. Most health facilities use the same ambient illumination in all areas. However, medical equipment could be de-emphasized by placing it in shadows, to be illuminated only when being checked. Track lighting could be used to emphasize the parts of the room that do not contain equipment. Patients might feel more at home with a bedside lamp that projects light out into the room and keeps the wall of medical equipment behind them in the dark. Visitors would also receive a less alarming impression if the patient were highlighted and the monitors, oxygen and suction connections, and IV stands were in the background. Variations in lighting could be an effective and relatively inexpensive way to reduce patient and visitor anxiety and decrease the imposing clinical look of most health-care facilities.

NOISE

Noise interferes with communication and productivity, increases irritability, and can cause pain or injury.[12] However, total silence can be discomforting also. Although people are capable of making some adjustments to a steady noise level, errors increase at the end of an 8-hour day. The ability to give patient instructions, to take the patient's history or other communications, and to communicate with managers are all impeded by high noise levels (85 to 90 decibels or more), and the effects compound with increasing frequency and duration of exposure to the noise.[13] Also, productivity increases and worker stress decreases as background noise levels decrease. Where it is not possible to design quieter work areas, sound-absorbing materials like drapes, carpets, and acoustical tiles should be used.

LOCATION

When considering location in the work environment, consider both department location and the designs within each department. Easy access for patients, workers, and equipment, and logical design are key, easy-to-use elements to implement in a work environment. Department location should be blatantly obvious to new patients and visitors. Signage should be large, distinct, bilingual (if necessary), and in Braille. Remember that people are more tense and anxious than usual when visiting a hospital, clinic, or other health-care facility. This anxiety may be reduced if patients or clients clearly understand how they are supposed to get to where they are going.

Good department location saves patient and employee travel time, reduces fatigue, and increases productivity. All emergency facilities should be close to one another. The emergency department, radiology department, and the laboratory should be close together.[14] In larger facilities, or when traditional grouping is not possible, satellite facilities should be considered. Having x-ray, respiratory care, and traction therapy stations on each floor or in each wing may prove more effective than large, centralized departments.

Department arrangement should be logical, with attention to coordinating traffic flow and minimizing worker fatigue.[15] Work materials should be available to the employees where they are needed so that they do not have to travel far for supplies they use routinely. Several small caches may be more effective than a centrally located supply room.

SPACE

Sufficient space in which to perform work is usually in short supply because of monetary constraints.[16] Employee personal space is another concern. Each employee should have some personal space, usually a locker, to call his or her own. There should also be space for employees to relax out of sight of patients and visitors. Last, there should be a place for employees to consult one another and their supervisors about concerns for patients.

LAYOUT

Frontline employees are often the best qualified to comment on the layout of department areas or rooms. Having to work with, and around, the equipment day after day often causes them to think about alternative designs. Many make changes if possible. Money spent on alterations is often well spent because layouts that are good for the employees and patients are usually good for productivity. The main consideration for layouts is having enough room to perform the required health-care procedures while minimizing the number of movements and the distance workers must travel.[17] Often a balance must be established between these two concerns. However, careful planning for each benefits the health-care facility and the health-care worker. The facility can experience greater productivity and the worker less fatigue.

EQUIPMENT

Equipment considerations include uniformity, age, ease of use, safety, and maintenance. Uniformity of equipment, although not always possible, can be an advantage. Errors decrease and productivity increases as the variety of equipment and sets of instructions decrease.[18] Although newer equipment requires some training and an adjustment period, employees often feel more confident and comfortable with equipment that looks new and still has all of its parts. Equipment that is easy to use reduces worker fatigue and increases efficiency while decreasing errors in patient treatment and time spent carrying out procedures.[19] All equipment must provide for worker and patient safety. Proper maintenance, the responsibility of the worker and management, can ensure that all of these conditions continue to be met.

SUPPLIES

Inadequate supplies lead to inefficiency, worker frustration, and decreases in the quality of patient care.[20] Not only must the quantity of supplies be adequate, but they must be where the workers need them, when they need them. One of management's more important functions is to make sure that employees have the resources to perform their jobs.

COLOR AND DECOR

The colors used in a health-care facility have an effect on employees and patients and consequently on the work performed. Colors should be selected that will be interesting for employees but not upsetting to the patients. Brighter and lighter colors are generally preferable to flat, drab medium hues. All color selections must be evaluated for their effect on the function of the department or room. Highly reflected, saturated colors, like gloss white or dark browns, which can alter the patient's color (and the patient's assessment) must be avoided.[21] Glare, especially in surgical areas, is also a concern.[22] Another functional concern is using different colors to identify different departments or areas. For example, having the nursing station or information area painted a contrasting color will help patients, visitors, and workers to locate it. Earth tones should be considered because they are not too bright or startling.[23] Also, because patients spend so much time supine, careful attention should be given to the ceiling. Finally, a balance should be obtained between colors that are interesting, colors that identify or provide information, and colors that contrast.

Decor can complement and augment color. As competition increases, health-care facility planners are paying more attention to decor for the customer's (patient's and client's) sake. As the shortage of health-care workers continues, this may also be the time to consider the decor that employees would like. Not only should the decor be clean, bright, and attractive, it should also be variable.

Employees should not only have input into the decor, they should also be free to contribute and change their surroundings. Flexible items like plants (real or silk), paintings, pictures, wall hangings, and even knick-knacks can be used. When the workers become tired of something, they should be able to trade or borrow new items.

A well-conceived decor can go a long way toward camouflaging the cold, clinical atmosphere of many health-care facilities. Maybe equipment could be painted something other than battleship gray or the other flat colors typical of health equipment. Improvements in decor for employees would also be beneficial for the patients. I remember touring a hospital in Las Vegas, Nevada, that looked more like a hotel than a hospital. Each room had its own balcony, and each floor had a different motif. It was a rather exclusive hospital, but the administrators had the right idea. And I do not remember their lacking for patients.

COMFORT

Employees, because they spend so much time on the job, should feel comfortable at work. Comfort is not limited to having a padded chair to sit on. The overall design and operation of the department or area should not be hectic or uncontrolled. Nor should employees feel that they are being constantly watched. In a department that I managed (but did not design), my office was directly across from the only area the workers had to gather in while waiting for their next patient. The office had a large window and a desk that only fit one way—facing the window. No matter what I did, it seemed as though I was watching them. This made some of them so uncomfortable that they would stand in the hallway or go around my office (and through the laboratory) to avoid the feeling that they were being observed. Finally I bought window blinds, which I kept closed. This helped somewhat, but a design with some thought toward the workers would have been better. The more relaxed and comfortable the employees feel, the better they perform.[24] The employees, patients, and management all benefit.

SECURITY

Security concerns go beyond the need for employees to be physically safe at work. Safety from harm at work and in the parking lot is important, of course.[25] However, employees also need to be safe from transmitted diseases, harmful chemicals, dangerous equipment, fire and electrical hazards, and radiation. Often it is not sufficient to have policies and procedures covering these hazards. Employees must know that policies exist and that they are adhered to. Properly maintained equipment is good not only for the client needing physical therapy and for the therapist; it is also a sign that there is concern for safety, a sign that speaks much louder than spoken or written words.

This is not to say that written policies concerning safety have no value. Written safety policies are indeed necessary, but they should be constantly reviewed with as much employee input as possible. As with the layout of work areas, frontline employees often have good ideas about methods that work because they handle these situations daily. Also, these policies should be communicated to other departments. All employees should know that they can walk past the radiology department or isolation ward without fear of radiation exposure or infection.

SOCIAL CONTACT

Behavioral management (see Chap. 5) theorists recognize that people work for many reasons, one of those being social contact. Although social contact is part of the working environment, planning that takes this into account is generally in short supply. The goal of the overall design should aid the social contacts that are a necessary part of each job and of the health professions. The design should provide for a measure of privacy, so that employees can speak with each other away from the patients and the public. The social aspects of work are part of the informal organization (see Chap. 5). At the least, the physical environment should not inhibit social contacts or unnecessarily isolate workers.

The Mental Work Environment

The *mental work environment* might also be called the psychological work environment. The mental work environment is the environment that you perceive. Its four main factors are the work itself, the managerial atmosphere, your coworkers' attitudes, and your attitude. This section will introduce these concepts, and they will also be dealt with in greater depth throughout the remainder of the book.

THE WORK ITSELF

The work itself has a major impact on the mental environment. It is composed of:

- The pace of the work
- The variability of the pace
- Duration of tasks
- Variety
- Concentration required
- Accuracy required
- Visibility of errors
- Level of responsibility
- Level of authority
- Level of autonomy

Most of these factors affect the mental environment by altering the stress level that you feel (Table 2–1).[26]

The Pace of the Work

The *pace* of the work refers to the time required to perform a job task and the time between each task. Some jobs are fast paced, with a very short interval between the end of one task and the beginning of the next, or involving a task that can (or must) be completed quickly. Others are slow paced, perhaps because of the time needed to prepare a room or equipment. Some jobs are slower paced because the diagnostic agents involved are slow acting or because the patient is just beginning therapy and

TABLE 2–1 • **FACTORS THAT AFFECT THE MENTAL WORK ENVIRONMENT**

Mental Work Environment Factor	Worker Control over Factor	Effect on Worker as Factor Increases
Pace of the work	Moderate	Stress increases.
Variability of the pace	Minimal	Stress increases.
Duration of tasks	Moderate	Boredom decreases; job satisfaction and performance increase.
Variety	Minimal	Interest and motivation increase.
Concentration required	Minimal	Fatigue and stress increase; accuracy and efficiency decrease.
Accuracy required	Minimal	Stress increases.
Visibility of errors	Minimal	Stress increases.
Level of responsibility	Higher	Stress increases.
Level of authority	Minimal	Stress decreases.
Level of autonomy	Moderate	Stress increases.

cannot move quickly. Generally, as the pace of the work increases, stress increases.[27,28]

The Variability of the Pace

Variability of the pace of the work refers to how steady the flow of work is. Some jobs have a steady, even flow. The pace may be fast or slow, but it is constant. These are most often jobs for which the time to perform the tasks is known and is relatively constant. In other jobs, the pace is highly variable, usually not controllable (although it may be somewhat predictable), and often described as "feast or famine."

In health care, patient flow is often the prime determinant of the variability of the work pace, although sometimes the equipment dictates the tempo. Magnetic resonance imaging (MRI) scanners and computed tomography (CT) scanners often have lower variability of pace. The equipment takes a certain known amount of time, and the throughput, as it is called, is fairly stable. Other times the service being performed can be controlled to decrease the variability, as in occupational and physical therapy. The emergency department is at the other extreme of the pace scale. Although there are certain trends (a rush from dinner time until about 10:00 P.M. during the weekdays), the volume is never really predictable, and the time to tend each patient is highly variable. Patient treatment needs can range from a sore throat to life-threatening accidents or gunshot wounds. In general, as the variability of the pace increases, stress increases.[29]

Duration of Tasks

Duration of tasks is defined as the time required to perform one job task. As the time required to perform a task decreases, boredom increases. As boredom increases, job satisfaction and performance decrease.[30] Typically, health-care workers do not suffer from this problem nearly as much as industrial workers. Some industrial tasks last from 3 to 5 seconds.

Variety

As the *variety* of tasks in a job increases, people's interest in their work increases. As interest increases, motivation increases.[31] But when a job is constantly repeated, it quickly becomes tedious. Task specialization usually yields high proficiency; however, everyone needs a change now and again. The worst case involves low variety and short duration of tasks. Not only is this boring, but safety, concentration, and productivity decrease in this situation. Jobs that have traditionally lacked variety should be expanded by making the worker responsible for a greater portion of a job or by adding tasks. This not only improves interest, but also helps reduce turnover.

Concentration Required

Different jobs and different tasks require varying levels of *concentration*. A high level of concentration that is sustained for a long time increases

BUILDING COMPREHENSION EXERCISE 2–2

Assessing the Mental Work Environment

Examine your current work environment. How much control do you have over each of these factors? How much does each factor affect you? For those factors that you can control and that have a negative effect on you, list actions you can take to reduce the negative effects.

Mental Work Environment Factors	Your Control over the Factor	How Factor Affects You	Actions You Could Take
Pace of the work	High level	Greatly increases stress	
	Moderate	Somewhat increases stress	
	Little or none	Minimal effect on stress	
Variability of the pace	High level	Greatly increases stress	
	Moderate	Somewhat increases stress	
	Little or none	Minimal effect on stress	
Duration of tasks	High level	Increases boredom	
	Moderate	Decreases job satisfaction	
	Little or none	Decreases performance	
		No negative effect	
Variety of tasks	High level	Decreases interest	
	Moderate	Decreases motivation	
	Little or none	No negative effect	
Concentration Required	High level	Increases fatigue and stress	
	Moderate	Decreases accuracy	
	Little or none	Decreases efficiency	
		No negative effect	

Exercise continues on following page 🧊🧊🧊

Accuracy required	High level	Greatly increases stress	
	Moderate	Somewhat increases stress	
	Little or none	Minimal effect on stress	
Visibility of errors	High level	Greatly increases stress	
	Moderate	Somewhat increases stress	
	Little or none	Minimal effect on stress	
Level of responsibility	High level	Greatly increases stress	
	Moderate	Somewhat increases stress	
	Little or none	Minimal effect on stress	
Level of authority	High level	Greatly increases stress	
	Moderate	Somewhat increases stress	
	Little or none	Minimal effect on stress	
Level of autonomy	High level	Greatly increases stress	
	Moderate	Somewhat increases stress	
	Little or none	Minimal effect on stress	

End of exercise. Text continues on following page.

fatigue, increases stress, and decreases accuracy and efficiency.[32] Whenever possible, tasks that require high concentration should be alternated with tasks that require lower concentration. There should also be a rough balance between the two. If it is not possible to alternate tasks with different concentration levels, then the number and the duration of rest periods should be modified to provide relief for the worker.

Accuracy Required

As the amount of *accuracy* required in a task increases, stress increases.[33] Many tasks in the health professions require 100 percent, or nearly 100 percent, accuracy. Surgical procedures, invasive diagnostic procedures, procedures utilizing ionizing radiation, and the dispensing of medications are all examples of tasks that have serious consequences for less than perfect performance. Technology is often employed in an attempt to improve performance by decreasing the reliance on people. Other options include ensuring that all equipment is in optimum working order, decreasing stress, decreasing fatigue, and combating boredom. Proper training is also vital when new equipment and procedures are introduced, and retraining can help employees maintain competency with difficult, complex, or infrequent duties.

Visibility of Errors

The *visibility* of an employee's errors affects stress levels. The more visible an error is to the patient, supervisor, or colleagues, the higher the pressure is to avoid errors. When a radiographer makes an error, the radiograph is hard evidence for all to see. The mistake can be seen, and it is obvious to coworkers, managers, and physicians. The patient also knows that something was wrong because he or she is brought back for an additional exposure. However, in most ultrasonography exams, inadequate scans are simply not recorded, and no one is the wiser.

Increased visibility of errors increases stress. This can be counteracted to a degree by the way in which associates and bosses handle mistakes. Gentle, constructive criticism produces greater results in most situations than does derision, insults, and harsh language. Likewise, you should be aware of how you handle mistakes you observe in others. If you point out the mistakes of others, and if you comment on all errors and ridicule people, you will make many enemies and must be prepared to be treated the same way by others when you make a mistake.

Level of Responsibility and Authority

Responsibility and authority should act in concert with each other. *Responsibility* means that you are held accountable for certain results. *Authority* means that you have been given the ability to fulfill your responsibilities. Problems and stress increase when someone has the responsibility for a task but management has not delegated that person the authority to carry it out.[34] For example, if you are given the responsibility for revising the procedures manual in your area but do not have the authority to make changes in the procedures, you will probably not be successful. Another example is being given the responsibility for improving the performance of students training for your profession. If you do not have the authority to make changes in their training program, you will have a difficult time fulfilling your charge. When responsibility is given without the requisite authority, stress and frustration increase, and productivity decreases or is nonexistent.

Level of Autonomy

As the *level of autonomy* required of workers increases, stress increases. However, this is usually a problem only when the workers have not been trained for autonomous activity.[35] Removing individual actions and decisions from work can be detrimental because this increases boredom and decreases productivity. Therefore, if the job requires that people work autonomously, then they must be trained to work independently and be given the authority to do so. They should then be held responsible for their actions. In addition, Fredrick Herzberg (see Chap. 9) and others[36] have said that such autonomy is not only a desirable part of every job, it is a necessary part. It is usually only when the job requires independent judgment or activity and the system or an overbearing boss does not permit it, that autonomy becomes a major problem for employees.

Most elements of the work's contribution to the mental environment affect stress and, consequently, productivity. Managers may evaluate each item for the positions they supervise and adjust them to minimize stress and maximize worker satisfaction and productivity. You can evaluate your current position, or a position you are contemplating accepting, and evaluate yourself in relation to the listed criteria. You may then look for the best match between the position you want and what is available.

THE MANAGERIAL ATMOSPHERE

The managerial philosophy has such a major impact on the mental work environment that all of Chapter 5 and much of Chapter 6 are dedicated to it. As a preview to those chapters, note that the major influences on the management atmosphere include the overall philosophy of the organization, the tasks you perform, and your immediate supervisor's style, level of management training, and experience.

COWORKER ATTITUDES

Volumes could be written about getting along with fellow workers, or the subject could never be discussed. Much depends on some basic assumptions that are made about work. There are many people who feel that the employees in a work group should, at the very least, be on civil, speaking terms with one another. These people recognize the social aspects of work. If they are managers, they are subscribing to the behavioral school of management (see Chap. 5). There are others who believe that employees are being paid to work—they are not being paid to like each other. This group of managers typically believes in the classical management style (see Chap. 5). How your coworkers feel and how you feel about this issue will affect the way you are treated, and, as will be seen in Chapters 6 and 7, the relationships found in the formal organization (or chain of command) and the informal organization (the social aspects of work) will also affect you.

What is important is finding a match between how you feel coworkers should be and how the others in a department feel. If you want to be part of a work group that goes out together outside of work, then you should look for a group that has a high level of camaraderie. If social interactions on the job are not important to you, then you may be more comfortable working alone (in a small clinic or hospital or on late shifts), or you may want to work in a large department where it is usually easier to do your work on your own without disrupting other social groups.

YOUR ROLE

No matter what shift you work, or where you work, eventually you will come in contact with other workers. Even if you work with others readily, the same things apply. People have bad days,

and things they say or do should not be taken too personally. This may sound simple, but too many people forget it or never learn it.

Everyone has a bad day once in a while. The reasons for this can be attributed to the stresses of work or to the demands of family and personal life. The causes are myriad. What is important is the way you react to your coworkers when they are having a difficult time. The key is to treat them the way you would like to be treated. You should use some of the compassion and empathy you have for patients with your coworkers. Specifically:

- Do not remind them of mistakes they have made.
- Be more available if they need help.
- Share a little of their workload.
- Don't complain if they don't do their "fair" share that one day.
- If they want to talk, be there to listen.
- If they do not want to talk, do not try to pry an explanation from them.
- Try to place them in a less stressful area for a day or give them easier, less taxing patients or assignments. This can be done by trading work for a day or, if you are in a supervisory position, by reassigning them that day.

If these things are done, everyone benefits. The person having difficulty benefits by having fewer items to deal with, and the patients and the employer benefit by placing the person in an area where he or she can perform with less stress and fewer mistakes. Even the other employees benefit by knowing that someone will look out for them when they are in a similar situation. All of this can prevent a bad situation from becoming worse.

Many people never think to include themselves as part of the mental work environment. In their view, the world acts on them—it is an external force that intrudes on them. They do not see themselves as a part within the world. They see themselves as an innocent beach with the external world crashing on them like waves. In the work environment everyone else makes up the mental atmosphere, and it affects them, but they are not a part of it. This is wrong. How you act contributes to the entire mental ecosystem and makes things better or worse for you. Much of this concerns communications and conflict management (see Chap. 3), but some comments concerning coworkers and managers are included here.

Possibly the two most important factors in coworker relations are to not take other people too seriously and to remember that everyone is human. These two would include being overly concerned with how much everyone else does, being paranoid, looking for hidden meanings in everything when there are none, and treating everyone with dignity.

Many people worry that other people are doing less work than they are—perhaps a leftover childhood concern related to worry that their brother or sister dried one fewer dish than they did. In fact, if some of these people spent half as much time doing their own jobs as they did worrying about what everyone else is doing, there wouldn't be any work left for anyone.

The main concern seems to be that everyone is getting paid about the same amount, so everyone should be doing the same amount of work. Many people feel that they have done a fair day's work if they did the same amount as everyone else. The standard is measured relative to other workers of the same type. This is wrong. A fair day's work is given for a fair day's pay. Pay comes from the employer. The employer judges the standard as to whether or not people gave a certain amount of work relative to the pay they received, not relative to what everyone else did. Work is judged in relation to pay, not in relation to other workers.

If everyone else in the department sits around, hides, or otherwise evades work, you are still obligated to do your job because you are being paid. At times this may be difficult to live with, but you should keep in mind that those who do not do their share, who do not live up to their end of the bargain with their employer, will be found out. Sometimes it takes a while, but their actions will be discovered, and they will pay a price. On the other hand, if you have pride in yourself and give your best effort despite what others are doing, this too will be noticed. You will be a valued employee whom employers will reward, promote, or fight to keep. You will be a professional employee.

Other employees appear to be paranoid when dealing with their coworkers. These are people who feel that others are always talking about them when they are not around. Some of them refuse to help their coworkers, feeling that helping others with make the others look better than they really are. As strange as this may seem, it happens even in the health professions.

Generally, health professionals work together in teams, assist one another, and publish journal articles so that all may benefit from an improved method. However, I have worked with people who would not give advice nor assist others. After observing these people for some time, I asked them why they didn't help their coworkers. One person said that he was not being paid to help others; he was paid just to do his own work. The others had a different answer—if they helped someone, that person would be as good as they were. Later, if they both wanted a promotion, they would have given up their "natural" advantage by helping the other person. When I said that participating as a team member, being part of the department, and assisting colleagues would go further in getting a promotion than any advantage gained by holding a small piece of technical knowledge, they remained unconvinced. In fact, they said that anybody could help their coworkers, even if they were just an "average" worker. I guess they felt that the little helpful hints they were keeping to themselves kept them above average. When I pressed them, they each said that they knew that when they were students, the teachers and practitioners always held back something so that they would always know more than the students!

It is difficult to understand this thinking. All health workers have a professional obligation to help one another for the good of the patients or clients. So do not be like these people. If you have to work with them, you still have a duty to help them, even if they will not help you. A professional employee does what is best for the patients or clients and the employer. A professional employee is above petty actions such as these and needs no reason to act professionally other than it is the professional thing to do.

There may also be coworkers who see hidden meanings in everything. For example, if every patient they are assigned to for a particular day is difficult, they take it to mean that the supervisor is angry at them. Or, if someone receives a promotion, they assume that person was promoted because the boss likes him or her, not because the person is qualified. These people may not realize that every patient that day was difficult or that the boss can only give one person a promotion. It is important to remember that it is very difficult and time-consuming to plot every action a person takes so that it carries a particular message. Usually this is more time than a boss has and requires far too much effort. If the boss gives you a particular assignment, it may be because you are the best one for the job, or because you were the first person he or she ran into. Do not take everything people do personally. It will be best for your mental health to take each assignment and immediately concern yourself with how you will complete it, rather than worry about why the supervisor picked you to do it.

If you want to have a more enjoyable work life, be more successful, receive more cooperation, and get along with your coworkers better, then treat everyone with dignity and respect. For some reason there are people who treat their patients like royalty but treat their coworkers like dirt. This is especially true if they feel the other worker is of lower status. *Everyone* should be treated the same. All should be treated the way you want to be treated. And if you think some other worker is beneath you, then picture your hospital or clinic without them. Picture a hospital with no cleaning personnel. Imagine a hospital without transporters. How would a hospital function without maintenance workers, nurses, respiratory therapists, accounting personnel, or medical lab technicians? Everyone in a hospital or clinic is vital to its survival. So everyone is entitled to be treated with courtesy and respect. Besides being the right thing to do, it is your professional responsibility to treat everyone the way you expect to be treated.

Summary

This chapter has discussed the physical and mental framework on which the work world is built. It has also laid the groundwork for the rest of this book. It has discussed how the physical work environment can affect work and has outlined items that you may wish to consider when looking for employment. The chapter has also introduced many topics that will be detailed in later chapters. Through this type of introduction you should notice how many sections of the working environment are interrelated. Notice how discussing coworker attitudes and your own attitudes is an almost arbitrary division. The mental environment

of your coworkers affects you, and your disposition affects your coworkers (Fig. 2–2). In return, your attitude affects how your coworkers treat you. The understanding of the interrelation and interaction of the various components of the working environment is one of the main goals of this book. You should concentrate on noticing this throughout the remaining chapters.

REFERENCES

1. Lowenberg, G, and Kelly, C: Current Perspectives in Industrial/Organizational Psychology. Allyn & Bacon, Needham Heights, Mass., 1998, p 427.
2. Stevenson, WJ: Production Operations Management, ed 6. Irwin/McGraw-Hill, Boston, 1999, p 323.
3. Fogarty, DW, et al: Production and Operations Management. South-Western Publishing, Cincinnati, 1989, p 72.
4. Stevenson, p 323.
5. Graf, D: Basic Building Data, ed 3. Van Nostrand Reinhold, New York, 1985, p 170.
6. Ibid, p 172.
7. Fogarty, et al, p 189.
8. Mahnke, FH, and Mahnke, RH: Color and Light in Manmade Environments. Van Nostrand Reinhold, New York, 1987, p 204.
9. Stevenson, p 323–24.
10. Mahnke, and Mahnke, p 151.
11. Ibid, p 157.
12. Stevenson, p 324.
13. Fogarty, et al, p 98.
14. Adam, EE, et al: Production and Operations Management, ed 5. Prentice-Hall, Englewood Cliffs, NJ, 1992, p 38.
15. Stevenson, p 324–25.
16. Fogarty, et al, p 124.
17. Stevenson, p 318–22.
18. Meredith, JR: The Management of Operations: A Conceptual Emphasis, ed 4. John Wiley & Sons, New York, 1992, p 341.
19. Ibid, p 279.
20. Mahnke, and Mahnke, p 184.
21. Ibid, p 193.
22. Goumain, P (ed): High-Technology Workplaces. Von Nostrand Reinhold, New York, 1989, p 45.
23. Fogarty, et al, p 306.
24. Meredith, p 341.
25. Steele, FI: Physical Setting and Organization Development. Addison-Wesley, Reading, Mass., 1973, p 101.
26. Herzberg, F: Work and the Nature of Man. World, Cleveland, 1966, p 36.
27. Karasek, R, and Theorell, T: Healthy Work: Stress, Productivity, and the Reconstruction of Working Life. Basic Books, New York, 1990, p 12.
28. McGregor, D: The Human Side of Enterprise. McGraw-Hill, New York, 1960, p 29.
29. O'Reilly, B: Is your company asking too much? Fortune, March 12, 1990, pp 38–46.
30. Herzberg, p 37.
31. Ibid, p 49.
32. Ibid, p 74.
33. McGregor, D, p 57.
34. Ibid, p 53.
35. Rothwell, WJ, and Kazanas, HC: Strategic Human Resource Development. Prentice-Hall, Englewood Cliffs, NJ, 1989.
36. Herzberg, p 51.

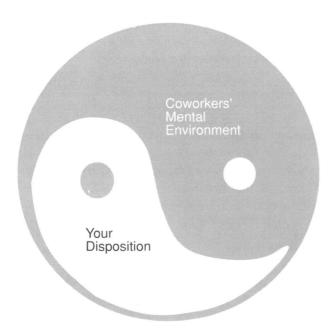

FIGURE 2–2 • The mental environment of your coworkers affects you, and your disposition affects your coworkers.

3 ◦ Communication: Verbal and Nonverbal

Objectives

On completion of this chapter, the reader will be able to:

☐ Differentiate between verbal and nonverbal communication.

☐ List and define the elements of nonverbal communication.

☐ List, define, and explain the contribution to communications that each of the three parts of a message makes.

☐ Define and explain the function of nonverbal communication.

☐ Identify types of nonverbal communication and explain the effect each has on communication.

☐ Describe communication styles that challenge managerial status along with those that acquiesce to it.

☐ List, define, identify, and explain common barriers to communication.

☐ List, define, identify, and explain methods for improving communication.

☐ Explain how the genders communicate differently.

☐ Define the basic types of conflict.

☐ Describe conflict management methods.

This chapter will concentrate on communication as it relates to coworkers and managers. Some topics may appear familiar to you if you have studied communications with patients or clients. Our purpose here, however, is to examine and improve communications among the health-care workers and managers.

Hopefully, improving communications with coworkers will reduce conflicts, make the entire organization more effective, and make your job easier and more enjoyable. In addition, an examination of nonverbal communications will make you aware of the messages you are sending to supervisors and of those you are probably expecting to receive. Such awareness should help you avoid learning these lessons the hard way—through experience, which often means you have already made a mistake. We will begin by surveying some general concepts in nonverbal communications.

Nonverbal Communication

IMPORTANCE OF NONVERBAL COMMUNICATION

Nonverbal communication is the use of gestures, facial expressions, and other inaudible expressions to transmit a message. Notice that the definition is "to transmit *a* message." It does not say "to transmit *your* message" or "to transmit your *intended* message." Frequently, people send conflicting verbal or nonverbal messages. As an example, consider the following health-care situation. A health-care worker is preparing to treat you or care for you. She asks you a series of history, or background, questions. At the same time she is busy placing the room in order, organizing paperwork, and adjusting equipment. What message do you receive? What do you feel she is more interested in—you or the physical environment? Do you get the impression that she cares about you? She may actually care about you a great deal, *but that is not what is being communicated.* Even if she were to state that she cared about you, you would probably not believe her. The exact same thing can occur between you and your coworkers or supervi-

sors. When your nonverbal message conflicts with your verbal message, the *nonverbal* message will be believed (actions speak louder than words).[1] If you are not aware of and do not attend to your nonverbal signals, you could unintentionally send the wrong message.

In *Silent Messages,* Dr. Albert Mehrabian[2] analyzes the messages people send. He divides messages into three parts: verbal, vocal, and nonverbal. The *verbal* part includes the actual words we use in a message. The *vocal* part of a message is the tone, or inflection, we place on those words. The entire message changes if we use a sarcastic tone rather than a sincere tone. The *nonverbal* part of the message includes the physical aspects—facial expressions, gestures, posture, eye contact. Mehrabian estimates that 7 percent of a message is verbal and 38 percent is vocal. That means that *55 percent* is nonverbal, and it contributes to each message in a number of ways (Fig. 3–1).

FUNCTION OF NONVERBAL COMMUNICATION

Nonverbal communication can complement, repeat, contradict, regulate, replace, or accent our verbal and vocal message.[3]

Nonverbal cues *complement* a message by adding reinforcement to what is said. Nonverbal cues that complement a message would not convey the message if used alone. Complementary cues support the intended message. An example would be the distance people stand from one another when talking. Generally, employees stand farther away from a boss than a coworker. To do so does not convey much of a message by itself (especially if they are facing away from each other), but when coupled with a friendly "Hello" in response to the boss's "Good morning," it does. It shows that you are responsive and respectful and that you are not challenging the boss's authority.

When a nonverbal cue adds to the verbal message but could also stand alone, it is *repeating* the message. For example, if someone told you some gossip, and you rolled your eyes as you said, "I *don't* believe it," you would be repeating your message. Either the nonverbal cue or the verbal

FIGURE 3–1 • Estimated importance of nonverbal, vocal, and verbal components of a spoken message.

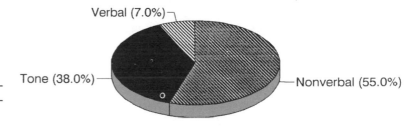

Verbal (7.0%)
Tone (38.0%)
Nonverbal (55.0%)

message could stand alone and still convey your disbelief.

Nonverbal cues can *contradict* verbal messages when they convey a meaning opposite to what is being said. Your look of boredom or distraction when the boss discusses the finer points of bulk-buying discounts and inventory control during lunch effectively negates your comment, "How interesting!"

Nonverbal communications can *regulate* a conversation by controlling the course of the discussion. For instance, touching someone's arm can send a signal that you wish to speak or that you wish to interrupt.

Substitution occurs when the nonverbal message replaces the verbal. Once again, actions speak louder than words. Substitution occurs when a boss gives someone an unwanted assignment, and instead of refusing or verbally protesting, the person stares coldly at the boss for a few seconds before turning to go perform the task.

Accenting differs from complementing in that accenting punctuates a part of a message, rather than lending general support to the entire message. Poking a finger into someone's chest is an example of accenting verbal communications.

These *functions* of nonverbal communication should be kept in mind as the types of nonverbal communication are discussed.

TYPES OF NONVERBAL COMMUNICATION

Physical Characteristics

A person's physical characteristics have a large impact on communications because we are highly visual creatures and because visual data are the most immediate information we receive about someone. Think of all the people you know and compare that number to the number of people on this planet. Of course, you know a very small percentage. However, as you are walking along, you can instantly recognize a known face in a crowd. You may not even know the person's name, but you will know whether or not you have seen him or her before. This is an amazing feat considering that all faces are essentially the same (two eyes, a nose, a mouth, and so on).

Although it is not always fair, it has been documented that people stereotype others based on immediate visual impressions. It has been found that people respond more favorably to people who are attractive, clean, well groomed, and well dressed.[4] This finding has three applications for you. First, remember it when applying for a job—many bosses base a major portion of the decision to hire a person on their initial visual impression. Second, be aware of these reactions from supervisors because they could affect your evaluations or chances for promotion. Third, consider that coworkers and clients or patients will respond more favorably to you if you are well groomed.

Other stereotypes have been found based on body habitus and size. You may be limited in the amount of influence you can exercise over your body style, but awareness of these assumptions may explain why certain people react the way they do. For example, many people identify overweight people as being more talkative, good-natured, dependent, and trusting. On the other hand, thin people are sometimes seen as more ambitious, tense, stubborn, pessimistic, and quiet. And some people feel that muscular people are more adventurous and mature.[5] Again, these perceptions are not always true and are not always fair, but such prejudices have been found to exist.

Clothing

Clothes not only affect the way others perceive us, but they affect the way we feel about ourselves. People with new, stylish clothes generally feel more comfortable. Clothes that do not fit well make people look uncomfortable, unkempt, and disorganized. Clothes that are dirty, worn, or wrinkled can give others the impression that you don't care about yourself.[6] Some then assume that if you don't care enough to look professional, you don't care enough to do professional work. Clothes can also communicate economic status, occupation, and values.

In applying this information to the work environment, keep in mind job interviews, reactions of superiors, and reactions of coworkers. When applying for a job, you should look professional. This does not mean that you have to wear a traditional white uniform, but you should look businesslike—neat and well groomed but not overdone. (Additional suggestions appear in Chap. 8.)

As mentioned previously with regard to physical characteristics, the way you dress could affect evaluations and promotions. Bosses may be hesitant to give a promotion to someone who dresses poorly, because doing so could send a message to other workers that such an appearance is acceptable.

Territoriality

People have individual and cultural preferences in their personal space; that is, the distance they like to keep others away from themselves—this depends on how they were taught in childhood, how well they know the other person, and the status of the other person.[7] In America, casual friends or acquaintances are usually kept 24 to 40 inches away. Personal friends are usually allowed within 6 to 18 inches. Intimate friends are allowed within 6 inches (as when someone is whispering to you).

Cultural differences associated with territoriality sometimes appear in the work world. In some cultures people stand much closer when speaking than is common in the continental United States. For example, Puerto Ricans often stand close together when conversing. To back away from them is considered rude.[8] This sometimes leads to a kind of dance that can cover quite a distance. One person moves in too close, the other backs away, and so on. Sometimes the person who prefers more personal space maneuvers a table between himself or herself and the other person. As a last resort, some people cross their arms in front of themselves, thus saving their last few inches of space.

In communication with managers, especially in America, people of higher rank expect, and are given, more personal space than people of lesser rank. When this is not possible, as in an elevator, tension results. Everyone in the elevator usually becomes silent and stares at the floor indicator panel.

The *relationship* between a manager and a subordinate can also be communicated through territoriality. To begin, being called to the manager's office means that, once there, you are on his or her turf. Being called to the manager's office, as opposed to the manager stopping by your work area, can indicate that the manager expects this to be a formal meeting. Managers may call you into their offices, and convey their higher status by expanding their territory: they may lean back in their chairs and put their feet up.[9]

Subordinates can also use territoriality to send messages. To sit somewhere other than in the designated chair or to remain standing would indicate a challenge to the manager's status or defiance to the manager's authority. Another way to challenge the boss would be to lean on or sit on his or her desk or to intentionally stand closer than normal. And, to many managers, the ultimate act of defiance would be for the subordinate to sit in their chairs.

Posture

Posture can be used to send a message or to read another person's intent. Postural nonverbal communication channels include body orientation, arm position, leg position, and general sitting posture.[10]

Face-to-face communication is what most bosses expect when speaking to subordinates. To do otherwise would be an act of defiance or anger. When in a group, *orienting* your body away from the group or boss shows that you are avoiding the situation or are trying to distance yourself from the group or conversation. When a boss addresses a group of workers, the employees usually form a semicircle in front of the manager. If the group leaves some space for others to join it, it is indicating its openness. If the body orientations do not allow for others to join, the group is conveying that it is closed to others.

When people cross their *arms* in front of themselves, they are showing a closed, or defensive, posture.[11] Approaching the boss with a request or a new idea when he or she is in this position could be a mistake. The same position, with a hand tapping the arm, conveys impatience or anger.[12] Better to approach this person later. Another arm position that can tell you not to approach someone is when the hands are grasping each other behind the back while the person is walking.[13] Generally this means the person is deep in thought, and you may not wish to break a manager's concentration just then.

Crossed *legs* convey a closed attitude just as crossed arms do. Legs draped over the arm of a chair or propped up on a desk may indicate a relaxed, casual attitude. More often these gestures are related to a feeling of superiority and are consanguineous to territoriality.

General sitting posture may convey messages also. Sitting behind a desk maintains territoriality and accents differences in status. On the other hand, some managers keep a round table in the office. Conferences are held at the table instead of the desk to promote openness and to de-emphasize status. Having a reclining chair allows a supervisor to lean back with his or her hands placed behind the head. This is meant to transmit superiority and an aggressive attitude.

I have seen two unusual approaches to posture communications. One manager had his chair adjusted so that he was higher than anyone sitting in the chairs in front of his desk. He said it allowed him to look down on everyone, reinforcing his rank (Lyndon Johnson did something similar in his presidential jet). The manager said he especially enjoyed having sales representatives in this position. He was convinced it allowed him to control the situation. Another person I worked with had no chairs in his office other than his own. He was an internal auditor at a hospital and was known for his toughness. He never explained why he did this, but I think the reason is obvious. It would be disturbing enough to be called to his office, but to then have to stand before him while being grilled about spending or documentation discrepancies must have made more than a few people hastily agree to what he said.

Facial Expression

The face is the most expressive area for nonverbal communications, and we spend a great amount of time looking at it during a discussion. The wide variety of emotions expressed through the face are a part of everyone's repertoire. To demonstrate this, try watching television with the sound off. It is amazing how well the story line can be followed.

Eye contact deserves special mention. Americans generally give more eye contact when listening.[14] In other words, a speaker only glances at the listener, whereas the polite listener looks at the speaker's eyes or face. However, a hard stare indicates anger, aggression, or defensiveness.[15] When a listener looks down at the floor while being accused of something, it is often taken as an admission of guilt.[16] We also tend to look away when asking an embarrassing question or one that makes us feel uncomfortable.

Keep in mind that there are cultural differences involving eye contact. In some cultures, especially Spanish-speaking cultures, looking down is a sign of respect.[17] In America the listener looks at the speaker more than the speaker looks at the listener; the speaker looks briefly at the listener and then looks away. In Britain the speaker gives more eye contact than the listener.[18] If a British manager and an American worker were talking to one another, they could be looking at each other and looking away from each other at exactly the wrong time for both of them.

Attention to your eye contact with managers and coworkers is important in order to send the desired nonverbal message. Higher-status people in America expect to receive more eye contact than they give. Conversely, less eye contact is given to someone whose position is below yours. Avoiding eye contact with a boss can signal indecisiveness or dishonesty, or it could be an attempt to avoid being noticed. Prolonged eye contact (staring) shows that you disagree with what the person is saying or that you are challenging the speaker's authority over you.[19]

Gestures

Hand gestures can almost be as expressive as facial gestures.[20] Anger can be communicated by making a fist or by a stab of an index finger into someone's chest. Throwing the hands and arms into the air can communicate exasperation. Arms crossed in front of the body shows a closed, or defensive, attitude. Confidence is sometimes shown with the hands placed on the hips. Wringing the hands displays nervousness. A person holding his or her earlobe sometimes shows hesitation. Careful attention to your hands and those of others would doubtless reveal even more.

Thus far the hand gestures mentioned have involved one person. Probably the most frequent polite hand gesture involving two people is the handshake. If someone offers you his or her hand so that it is perpendicular to the floor, a neutral attitude is being conveyed. A hand with the palm facing down indicates that the person feels that he or she is dominant. This is also true if the hand starts vertical (neutral) and then is turned so that it is on top of yours. On the other hand (no pun intended), a person with the palm facing up is revealing an open and cooperative attitude.[21] The slight palm-up offering should be the one used with your boss when you do not wish to challenge his or her position or authority.

Verbal Communication

COMMUNICATION PROCESS

Each message contains more than words, as seen in the previous section on nonverbal communication. Furthermore, each message is affected by three things:

1. The meaning the sender puts on the message
2. The meaning the receiver puts on the message
3. Interference, or noise, between the sender and the receiver[22]

In other words, you may mean one thing, but someone may interpret it in another way.

The sender of a message always imparts a meaning with that message. As has been mentioned, this meaning may be supported or contradicted by nonverbal communication. The meaning may also be changed by the tone used. For example, words that would appear sincere on paper can be made to sound cruel or biting by using sarcasm. Meaning can be altered depending on which word in a sentence is accented. And sometimes what is not said is more important than what is said.

The receiver also affects the message. He or she may disbelieve most of what is being said—and thereby not believe your intended message. The receiver's attitude or emotional state may alter your message. Someone who is tired or has had a difficult day may treat any conversation as irritating. Or a person having trouble at home may greet

Communication: Verbal and Nonverbal

a coworker's friendly "Good morning!" with a gruff "What's so good about it?"

Interference, or noise, is anything that obstructs the communication process. It can range from the noise created in a busy workplace to the noise imparted by the communication channel itself. For instance, there are five communication channels common to the workplace:

- Written communication
- Telecommunication
- Third-party communication
- Face-to-face communication
- Group communication[23]

Written communication includes letters, FAXs, e-mail, and memos. Some managers feel that communicating to others in this manner assures that the intended message will come across. The managers reason that everyone will read the same words and therefore everyone will get the same message. However, the actual words amount to only 7 percent of a message. The remainder is composed of 38 percent tone and 55 percent nonverbal cues.[24] Also, the manager may have the same words in the memo, but because 93 percent of the message is missing, the receiver is freer to place his or her own inflection and interpretation on them (Fig. 3–2). In addition, written communications do not allow for immediate interaction. If the receivers have questions, they cannot ask them at that moment. They may even have to respond in writing or otherwise have a considerable delay in receiving an answer.

E-mail is best for shorter messages—two pages is stretching the limit. If you have a longer message, then send it as an attachment. E-mail messages should contain only information that you would feel comfortable allowing everyone to read because it is possible for employers to monitor (read) e-mail messages, and even retrieve deleted messages. When typing an e-mail, don't type everything in capitals; it appears that you are shouting at people. Don't use abbreviations; not everyone is familiar with them. Finally, don't assume that everyone in the organization uses e-mail. If you need to know that someone received your message, set the Return Receipt function, which will send you a message when the recipient has accessed your message.

Telecommunication includes telephones, intercoms, and other voice communications. These can be more effective than written communication because they use 45 percent of a message's capability (7 percent verbal and 38 percent tonal), and they allow for immediate interaction for the receiver and the sender (Fig. 3–3). However, the majority of a message's potential is still not available to the receiver.

On the surface, third-party communication may seem to offer the least noise because verbal, tonal, and nonverbal information is available. In fact, it is the worst of the four. Not only does the message have the meaning the sender intended, it is also subject to a second meaning—that of the person acting as the communication channel. That message may be, *or may not be,* what the sender intended.

Face-to-face discussions are best. They offer the full range of communication: the sender can impart the desired meaning, and the receiver can ask questions or ask for clarification of meaning if necessary. Face-to-face communication is best for delivering the maximum amount of information with your message, but it may not always be the most practical method. Group communication can be very useful especially when the same message needs to be delivered to a number of people and those people may have similar questions, or when there are problems to be solved or ideas to be generated. The attention of the sender is divided among the group members, however, rather than being focused on one individual as it is in face-to-face communication. Therefore, communication channels and interference can be ranked in order of effectiveness as:

1. Face-to-face communication
2. Group communications
3. Telecommunication
4. Written communication
5. Communication via a third party

Note that these rankings are determined according to which channel delivers the maximum amount of the message, allows for immediately feedback, and focuses the attention of the sender and the receiver (Table 3–1).

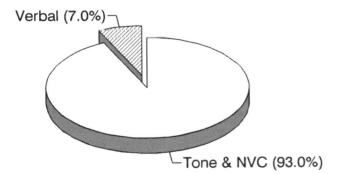

FIGURE 3–2 • Estimated importance of tone/nonverbal and verbal components of a written message.

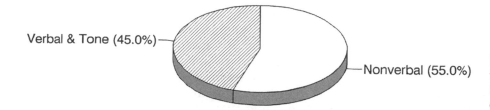

Verbal & Tone (45.0%)

Nonverbal (55.0%)

FIGURE 3–3 • Estimated importance of verbal/tonal and nonverbal components of a telecommunication message.

BARRIERS TO COMMUNICATION

In addition to the communication channel, a number of other barriers interfere with effective communication. These factors do not influence messages as much as they prevent communication from occurring. They include lying, prejudice, closed words, judging, attacking the person, snap judgments, and rank.

Lying can be defined as deliberately deceiving others to their loss or for your gain. Obviously this is a barrier to communication. Even though it would be quite helpful, there is no method to detect all liars all of the time. There are certain signs that can indicate whether or not someone is lying, but some are so subtle that it is almost impossible to consciously look for them.

We sometimes subconsciously notice clues pointing to people's lying. For example, the eyes can indicate lying through eye contact, blink rate, and pupil dilation. Many people believe that liars are unable to maintain eye contact for long. Accomplished liars, however, are quite good at this because it is relatively easy to control. However, blink rate and pupil dilation are not easy to control. People who are lying may blink more often than people who are telling the truth. Pupil dilation is virtually impossible to control, but it is hard to see. A high state of emotional arousal, which oc-

curs when someone is lying, causes the pupils to enlarge.

More easily observable indicators of possible lying include blushing, sweating, and facial expression. Some people cannot help but blush or sweat when they are lying or hiding something, especially when they are embarrassed or when telling a big lie. However, certain people blush just from being talked to and sweat for other reasons. Facial expressions may indicate lying when the expression is held longer than normal (which is 1 second) or when the expression begins after the spoken words it goes with (genuine expressions occur with the words or even a little before they are spoken).

Remember that these signals just show the possibility that someone may be lying. They do not prove lying. Also, because some of these signals are very subtle, we sometimes find that we feel uneasy about what someone says. This may be because we are registering these signals subconsciously, or it may be because we are misinterpreting the message.

Prejudice, prejudging, prevents communication from happening when a person assumes something will be true before it actually happens, as in the following example: "I have dealt with doctors before, and they were arrogant. You are a doctor; therefore, you will be arrogant." Well, *some* doctors are arrogant, but so are some people in every occupation. That does not mean the next doctor

TABLE 3–1 • COMMUNICATION CHANNELS AND THEIR USES

Communication Channel	When to Use the Channel
Face-to-Face	Whenever possible. For sensitive or confidential communications. When feedback is needed, especially to explain complex or confusing information.
Group	When the same important message would be delivered to many and they might have questions. When input from many areas is needed.
Phone	When something is urgent—so urgent there is no time for face-to-face communication. When the parties are separated. When the message is brief and an answer or confirmation is needed. When the message can be adequately conveyed without nonverbal communications.
Written	When the message is brief, easy to understand, and must be disseminated to many people, as with an announcement. When documentation is needed. When a reminder message needs to be sent to many.
Third-Party	Rarely, if ever.

you meet will be. Also, even if it were true that most doctors are arrogant (and I do not mean to say that they are), it still does not mean that the next one will be. There are always exceptions. Prejudice, then, is unfair. It is unfair to you in that it may keep you from communicating with, or from getting to know, others. It is unfair to the other person in that he or she may be judged and treated wrongly. Another problem is that people guilty of prejudice may make their beliefs into self-fulfilling prophecy. They may allow prejudice to taint the message to fulfill their belief. For example, I have heard people say, "I've worked with students before, and they slow me down too much." If they are assigned a student, they may then convince themselves that the student is responsible for any delays, or they may say, "See, I could have been done with this if not for this student." They can't prove this, of course. They would have to repeat the same procedure with the same patient and time both performances to prove the point. Barring such proof, they assume their biased opinion to be true.[25]

Closed words—for example, *all, none, everyone,* and *never*—are exclusionary. They eliminate other possibilities. They inhibit communication when used as part of generalizations, as in, "They *never* get the patient here on time," "*All* of the people on that shift are lazy," or "They're *always* rough with the clients." Not only would it be rare for statements like this to be true, but it would prevent communication by evoking a defensive response from the subject of each of them. Few people would not be defensive if told that they "*always* act unprofessionally."[26]

Judging interferes with communication when it masquerades as reporting. Judging means that a value judgment, an evaluation, of something is made. The thing is good, bad, better, or best. Reporting separates fact from opinion. Saying that an employer pays "poorly" tells us little. What is "poor" to one person (maybe someone with 10 years' experience) may be acceptable to another (someone right out of school). Saying that an employer's starting salary is $14.00 per hour is reporting a fact. The receiver is then free to make his or her own judgment on the adequacy of the pay.[27]

Attacking the person refers to assailing the entire person, rather than limiting comments to his or her behavior. Saying "I can't stand *him*. He's so slow" is attacking the person. Saying "I don't like that it takes him so long" talks about his behavior. Attacking the person requires someone to change on a fundamental level. Criticizing behavior requires people to change only one small part of themselves.[28]

Snap judgments, or premature closings, result when people make decisions based on first impressions or based on limited information (jumping to conclusions). Some people make snap judgments based on appearance or based on their first experience working with someone. They then extrapolate that behavior and judge the entire person. I have worked with a number of people who were absolutely convinced that they could tell if a person was going to be a good health professional or would successfully complete an educational program after only a few minutes of an interview. They would then point to the few times they were right as verification of the person's abilities—they would ignore the many times they were wrong. Some snap judgments are harmless, as in those times when we instantly "hit it off" with a new coworker. It is when snap judgments are negative that they are the most harmful and wrong.[29]

Rank refers to a person's position or status. It is a barrier to communication when it prevents a person of one rank from talking openly to a person of another rank. It is very common. One form that is frequently seen is when people of lower rank are reluctant to report problems to people of higher rank. However, it is also seen in the awkward conversations people at the top of an organization have with those at the bottom of the organization. In this case the conversation may turn to the weather or other harmless topics, with little or no real communication about the organization ever taking place. Here the high-ranking people are often just as uncomfortable communication as are those of lower rank.

IMPROVING COMMUNICATION

The first step to improving communications is to want to change. You must admit that change is possible and that it is desirable. Second, objectively look at the way you communicate with others. Identify which of the barriers to communication affect you. Third, actively try to change. You must constantly look for chances to improve your communication. Fourth, realize that there is a difference between hearing and listening. *Hearing* occurs when sound hits your ear and is translated to your brain. *Listening* occurs when you actively attend to this information. Most people can hear; fewer can listen. Fifth, you must realize that, like many things, this change probably will not come easily. It is not impossible to improve your communications, but it will require some effort. (This is the step where many fail—too many people want instant, painless results.) Beyond this initial commitment, here are some further suggestions.

Never fake attention. No communication can take place if you are not listening. Instead,

BUILDING COMPREHENSION EXERCISE 3–1

Improving Your Communications

Complete the following exercise to become a better communicator.

Evaluate Your Communication Style

1. How often do you tell significant lies?

    1. Rarely

    2. Monthly

    3. Weekly

    4. Daily

    5. Hourly

2. How often do you jump to a conclusion before knowing all the details or before something actually happens?

    1. Rarely

    2. Monthly

    3. Weekly

    4. Daily

    5. Hourly

3. When do you form an opinion about someone?

    1. After knowing them quite a while

    2. After your second meeting with them

    3. Within the first minutes of meeting them

    4. The moment you meet them

    5. Before meeting them

4. How often do you use words like *always, everyone, no one, all, never, everything,* and *nothing* while complaining about things or commenting about others?

    1. Rarely

    2. Monthly

    3. Weekly

    4. Daily

    5. Hourly

Exercise continues on following page 🔲🔲🔲

5. When listening to people, how likely are you to disregard what they say because they look different than you or look different than you think they should?

    1. Very likely

    2. Somewhat likely

    3. Neither likely nor unlikely

    4. Somewhat unlikely

    5. Very unlikely

6. If you know of a problem in your work area involving another person, how likely are you to tell your boss about the problem?

    1. Very likely

    2. Somewhat likely

    3. Neither likely nor unlikely

    4. Somewhat unlikely

    5. Very unlikely

7. How likely are you to interrupt others when they are talking?

    1. Very likely

    2. Somewhat likely

    3. Neither likely nor unlikely

    4. Somewhat unlikely

    5. Very unlikely

8. How often do you *pretend* to listen to what others are saying?

    1. Never

    2. Rarely

    3. Occasionally

    4. Often

    5. Routinely

9. When you don't understand what someone is saying, how likely are you to ask them to clarify what they said until you do understand?

    1. Very likely

    2. Somewhat likely

    3. Neither likely nor unlikely

    4. Somewhat unlikely

    5. Very unlikely

Each question refers to a particular communication problem (see below). If you answered 4 or 5 to any questions, you *should* work to improve that area. If you answered 2 or 3 to any questions, you *could* work on improving these areas. If you answered 1 to any questions, you probably do not have any problems in those areas.

Exercise continues on following page ❧ ❧ ❧

Question 1 was concerned with lying; Question 2, prejudice; Question 3, snap judgments; Question 4, using closed words; Question 5, attacking the individual; Question 6, rank; Question 7, interrupting; Question 8, faking attention; and Question 9, not verifying a message.

List areas that you should or could improve here.

_____

_____

_____

_____

_____

Reread the corresponding section in the text and list specific methods you could use to improve each area listed above.

_____

_____

_____

_____

_____

Track the number of times each week that you use each improvement method. After 1 month answer questions 1 through 9. Identify areas that are improved and areas that need further improvement.

End of exercise. Text continues on following page.

concentrate on what the speaker is saying (not on distractions or on his or her appearance), and don't get so emotional that you stop hearing and start formulating a response. Hear the speaker out. Do not interrupt.[30]

When you are unsure of a speaker's message—when you are not clear about what he or she meant—ask. In many work situations, it is too important to leave a message partially understood. Paraphrase what you thought you heard. Verify the message so that you know what was meant, in no uncertain terms. Repeat the message back to the sender. Ask. Say things such as, "Are you saying . . .?" or "Just so I'm clear on this . . ." or "What I'm hearing is. . . Is that what you meant?"[31,32]

Gender Differences

Men and women communicate differently.[33] That is not to say that one gender communicates better than the other; they simply communicate differently. Unfortunately, the differences often lead to miscommunication. Gender is only one of numerous ways communications are influenced, because not every person communicates the same way. People have tendencies, and there are many exceptions, but to improve communications, we must start somewhere. So we begin with the tendencies researchers have discovered.

MEN

Men communicate according to an unstated hierarchy.[34] Men evaluate each communication to determine whether they were superior or subordinate in the exchange; they do not like to be subordinate.[35] It is as if they are playing king-of-the-hill. Giving men orders, giving them unasked-for advice, or questioning their ability or competence are ways that make men think they are subordinate. How then do men survive in organizations without constantly fighting for power? Certainly, some are always fighting for power. Many others do not openly fight for the organization's power because men can live with different power levels if the levels are clear and accepted. However, many times the struggle to be superior comes out in other ways. A man may do what his boss says while thinking that he is superior in other ways (he is younger, is stronger, or has a faster car).

Another method men use to determine who is superior and who is subordinate is to make challenging statements that are forceful and definite. He determines whether or not he is superior and correct by the kind of argument others give him. If no one challenges his statement, or if the challenge is weak, he will conclude from this that he is correct!

Men also consider themselves to be problem solvers. Usually they like to solve problems alone without anyone else's advice. Giving a man advice when he hasn't asked for it is the same as telling him he is not capable of handling a situation, which means he now feels subordinate and the advice giver is superior.[36] Besides living in their hierarchies, men gauge their success according to the results they achieve.[37] Question or take away their achievements, and they feel they have failed.

When men encounter someone else's problem, they present a solution. When men don't have an answer, or when they are facing increased stress, they become more introverted.[38] When stressed or facing a difficult problem, men can become intensely focused. They withdraw into themselves until the problem is solved or until the stress is reduced. This can be difficult for women to handle because they want to offer help and talk about the problem to the same extent that men do not wish to talk.

Another characteristic of male communications is the tendency of men to take words literally.[39] If someone asks a man if he wants to do something, he may very well say "no." If the person then says, "You mean you wouldn't do this for me?" a man will often reply, "Sure, I'll do it, but that isn't what you asked me. You asked me if I wanted to it; I don't want to, but I will anyway." Notice that not only is the man taking the words literally, but now, by doing something he has said he doesn't want to do, he is doing the other person a favor, and is therefore showing his superiority in this situation.

Space does not permit a complete investigation of male communications, but these examples are representative and at least serve to point out the major considerations when communicating with men. This also serves as a fair, if brief, introduction to contrast how male communications differ from female communications, as you'll see in the following section.

WOMEN

Women, unlike men, are not typically concerned with hierarchies. Instead, women tend to have one close friend.[40] Rather than try to determine who is superior, women tend to comfort and console one another in their conversations.[41] Typically, it is more important to women to share feelings and support one another.[42] To show support and understanding, women relate similar experiences. Rather than offer a solution to a problem, as a man would, women offer empathy. Offering a solution to a woman's concern can be seen as negating or dismissing her feeling.[43] Women want empathy, not solutions.[44]

Of importance in the workplace is that women tend to soften and qualify what they say rather than give orders.[45] As a means of softening things and making them less harsh, women use generalities and metaphors.[46] Women often make suggestions, rather than give directions.[47] This is not necessarily an advantage in a workplace with men because it is sometimes seen as a sign of weakness or indecision and is not the strong challenge that men look for.[48]

In high-stress situations, women tend to feel overwhelmed.[49] They will then often seek out others so that they can unburden themselves.[50] When frustrated, women tend to use closed words like *all, everything,* and *never* to express how they feel (as in "I *never* get any help" or "Why do I have to do *all* the work?").[51] At these times, they do not mean for others to take them literally.

IMPROVING GENDER COMMUNICATIONS

What can be done to improve communications between the genders? First, try not to view the other gender's style through your own gender's style. For example, men need to understand that women soften orders but still mean for them to be followed, and women need to understand that men take things literally so they should state what they really mean. Second, learn more about how the other gender communicates and try to adjust your communications accordingly. Third, watch the reactions of others to ensure they receive the message that you sent. Fourth, watch what others say to you and notice your reactions to what is said. Are you receiving the message they are sending? Other, more specific suggestions are in Tables 3–2 and 3–3.

TABLE 3–2 • SENDING MESSAGES TO MEN

Suggestions for Talking to Men	Rationale
Ask, do not order, men to do things.	Ordering men makes them feel subordinate; if you ask them, they feel they are doing you a favor and they feel superior.
Challenge men when they make declarations.	Men determine who is correct according to the challenges they receive.
Don't give men free advice.	Men solve problems alone. If they need help or advice they will ask; giving them free advice is the same as telling them they can't do it.
Ask what you really want to know.	Men take things literally, so don't hint at things.
Don't use closed words like *always* or *never*.	Men take things literally; using closed words makes it sound as if they are being blamed and this makes them defensive.

TABLE 3–3 • SENDING MESSAGES TO WOMEN

Suggestions for Talking to Women	Rationale
Listen.	Women often need to just share their feelings.
Soften orders and directions; use suggestions rather than orders.	Women communicate less directly and often generalize.
Don't give only answers and solutions.	Giving an answer when none was sought negates a woman's feelings.
Show empathy and discuss experiences you have had that are similar to hers.	Women view this as support. A woman's sense of self is largely derived from the quality of her relationships.
Give details along with the summary.	Women are good at seeing details; they look for and expect them.
Look beyond a woman's literal words to find out what she really wants to communicate.	Women speak in generalities and metaphors; they often hint at things.

BUILDING COMPREHENSION EXERCISE 3–2

Enhancing Communication between Genders

You need to communicate the following messages. Rephrase each message as if you had to address a woman, and then a man. Compare the two versions. Are they different? How are they different? Should they be different according to the discussion on gender communications?

The person needs to be less rude with coworkers from other departments.

For a woman _____

_____

_____

For a man _____

_____

_____

The person is needed to work overtime.

For a woman _____

_____

_____

For a man _____

_____

_____

The person needs to take less time to complete each procedure.

For a woman _____

_____

_____

For a man _____

_____

_____

End of exercise. Text continues on following page.

General Employee Communications

Traditionally, managers have stressed *downward communications*. These communications come from high-ranking people and are distributed down the chain of command. However, some managers have been trying to improve *upward communications*—those that start with frontline workers and travel up the chain of command. More than ideas stuffed in the suggestion box, this feedback is seen as a valuable method of improving the organization and taking the pulse of the company.

Many employees, when asked formally for feedback, have nothing to say. However, when the meeting is over and the boss is gone, they have plenty of complaints. Some reluctance to speak is because of the fear of a boss's higher rank. People seem hesitant to talk openly in front of authority figures. It is thus mainly up to the boss to break down this barrier and get to know the workers until they feel more like they are talking to a peer. Some reluctance may be attributed to the newness of the boss's asking for information rather than telling people what to do. And some is because workers believe that even if they do mention a problem, nothing will be done to solve it. However, if the workers ever want to have a say in the organization, they need to say something when asked.

Look at the situation from the manager's point of view. Let's say that, as the manager, you have brought the department personnel together to find out where you can help them the most in completing their work. You ask and get essentially no reply. After the meeting breaks up, you hear rumors that some people in the department did in fact have something to say. So you try again next week. You point out your willingness to help. You try to get them to talk. You point out that "the squeaky wheel gets the grease." The meeting results in few comments because the workers feel "the squeaky wheel gets replaced first." How many times do you keep on asking? How many times do you go to a dry well?

If managers ask, you must give them an answer. If you don't, they will stop asking. They will not keep putting forth effort without getting some results in return. Neither would you. If you want to improve communications, if you want to have a say in the way things are done, then you must show the manager that it is worthwhile to take the time to get your opinion.

MEETINGS

Meetings are one of the most common forms of employee communication. Meetings need to be well planned or they can waste massive amounts time and frustrate those in attendance. A poorly planned and conducted meeting does nothing to further the organization's goals. On the other hand, sessions that are properly planned and led can generate more solutions, better solutions, and give more people a voice in the decision-making process. There are six main considerations to take into account when organizing a meeting.

Have a Clear Purpose

Only call a meeting when there's a good reason to have one so you don't waste people's time. Never call a meeting just because you think it has been a while, and never call a meeting when what you have to say could be covered in a memo or an e-mail. Good reasons to call a meeting include your needing to present the same complicated information to many people, when a number of people need the same information and they are likely to ask questions, or when you need a group to solve a problem. When you have the responsibility for calling a meeting, be certain that you have a planned agenda. An agenda can preventing wasting time and can ensure that no topics are accidentally missed.

Consider How Many to Invite

For practical purposes the number of people at problem-solving and discussion meetings should be about five to seven. If too few are invited, there may be too little variety of ideas; if too many are invited, the discussion is much more difficult to manage, some people may not speak up, and there is the chance for smaller factions to break off from the main group and work against the purpose of the group or conduct disruptive side discussions. If the meeting is a presentation followed by a question-and-answer period, many more people can be invited. In this case, inviting more people may save time. For instance, one person may ask a question that 23 others also thought of, and you will only have to answer it once for all of them.

Be Aware of the Clock

Set exact times for meetings to begin and end. Don't schedule open-ended meetings because they tend to drag on and on. Be sure to start and end the meeting on time. If you use all of your scheduled time, you can then decide whether to extend the meeting or schedule another. Another reason to set exact times is that it shows respect for other people's schedules and allows them to better organize the rest of their day. When planning the length of a meeting, consider setting the meeting for 1 hour or less. If the meeting must go longer, plan for breaks and moving around. Remember, the brain can only absorb what the butt can endure. Once people's bottoms go numb, you've lost them.

Keep the Meeting Brief

Send out the agenda and all materials that can be read before the meeting. If you will be asking people to contribute ideas, encourage them to come to the meeting with some already prepared and copied. Only do what must be done in the presence of everyone.

Think about Physical Surroundings

The meeting room arrangement can have a major effect on the people attending the meeting. For example, those who sit at the ends of the conference table are frequently perceived as having more power and influence than those who sit on the sides. People sitting side-by-side tend to have more difficulty seeing and communicating with each other. Tables designed so that everyone appears to be in an equal position, such as round tables, tend to encourage the free flow of ideas and discourage the domination of a meeting by one individual. Be aware of the temperature, ventilation, lighting, and equipment needs for each meeting. Hot, stuffy rooms can put people to sleep. If there are no shades for windows, it may be impossible to use an overhead projector or PowerPoint presentation. Always be familiar with the room you are using or check it out in advance to avoid looking incompetent.

Clearly Identify Everyone's Responsibilities

Another way to waste the potential a meeting has for success is to fail to make clear what people need to do. To make this task easier for you, do the following:

- Always prepare an agenda and if necessary send it to everyone before the meeting.
- Obtain information that can help with the meeting's results.
- Make sure everyone participates; if you invited people to solve problems then make sure you get their opinions.
- Decide on follow-up actions. Determine each person's follow-up responsibilities and make sure the person clearly understands what they are.
- Finally, make sure the follow-up actions are carried out.

AGENDAS

There are two main types of agendas—planned and hidden. Meetings called to provide information or to find a solution to a problem typically have a planned agenda. There is generally a good idea of what should be covered during the meeting. The planned agenda is useful in that it serves to guide the group's activities toward a pre-established goal. A planned agenda can help conserve scarce and valuable time. When preparing a planned agenda, first write down all of the topics that need to be covered, then organize them in a logical order. After they are organized, estimate the time each item will take and determine the length for the meeting.

Although you may prepare a planned agenda, there is the possibility that one or more people will have a hidden agenda. A hidden agenda is basically the attitudes and feelings that a person brings to a meeting. The hidden agenda may be thought out in advance of the meeting, or it may suddenly emerge. In some instances, people with hidden agendas try to block the planned agenda. When conducting a meeting, you should try to prepare for hidden agendas and then keep them from moving the meeting too far from its original course.

HELP IN GENERATING IDEAS DURING A MEETING

There are two useful and easy-to-use techniques for generating ideas or solutions during a meeting—brainstorming and brainwriting. During brainstorming, group members express themselves freely, regardless of how crazy or wild their ideas may appear to the other group members. The usual guidelines for brainstorming sessions are that:

- Everyone is encouraged to participate.
- A large number of ideas are to be generated.
- Group members listen to and build on others' ideas.
- Wild, creative ideas are encouraged.
- The atmosphere is free from criticism or evaluation.
- No idea or thought is squelched by either the idea's originator or the group members.
- All presented ideas are recorded.

Brainstorming sessions have proven helpful in generating a large number of potentially useful ideas. In a freewheeling session, useful ideas tend to build on less useful ones. If the group is large or if some people, for whatever reasons, are reluctant to contribute out loud, you should consider a second technique—brainwriting.

This small-group, idea-generating technique also ensures everyone's participation, and it can sometimes be used before a meeting. As with brainstorming, people build on each other's ideas, but before discussing ideas, each person writes his or her ideas on a piece of paper. Papers are then placed in the middle of the table and each is randomly examined. People then try to build on the presented ideas. Brainwriting offers some significant advantages over brainstorming. With brainwriting:

- The activity of writing tends to result in more complete and better thought-out ideas.
- Domination of the idea-generating process by a few members is less likely.
- Socializing and wasting time are more difficult.
- Emotionally charged or controversial topics can be handled more easily.

Both brainstorming and brainwriting are valuable, although brainstorming may be more valuable when the people in the group have different knowledge (as when each person is from a different department), and brainwriting may be more valuable when everyone has similar knowledge (as when each person is from the same department).

Conflict Management

Sometimes it seems that whenever two or more people are gathered together, there will be conflict. Conflict does not have to be bad, however. Conflict can be positive or negative, depending on how it is handled. The amount of conflict can vary, depending on your style of communicating. And, it may not be possible to solve every conflict, but it is possible to manage it so that it can be lived with.[52]

Conflict can be positive or negative—the decision is up to those in conflict. A *negative conflict experience* results when one or both sides view the situation as having the following characteristics:

- Us-against-them distinctions are felt.
- An all-or-nothing attitude is dominant.
- Each side sees only their point of view.
- Conflict is personalized.

In contrast, a *positive conflict experience* is more likely to result when both sides feel the circumstances to have these features:

- We-versus-the-problem attitude.
- Work is toward mutual satisfaction.
- Mutual needs are recognized.
- Discussion centers on facts and issues.[53]

A mutually agreeable result is more likely to come about if the people in the conflict view the *problem* as the focus of the conflict. The negative alternative is for each side to see the other as the enemy. In such a situation, one side wins and the other side loses, or both sides lose—it is rare for both sides to win in this way.

When both sides see the other as the enemy (instead of seeing the problem as such), the tendency is to try to gain everything. The feeling is to work for total victory. Too often the result is total defeat. The alternative is for both sides to work toward a mutually satisfying solution (by viewing the problem as the problem, and not each other).

To most effectively work for a mutually satisfying end to the conflict, both sides must be able to see the other point of view and to realize that there are mutual needs. If each side sees theirs as the only view—that their opinion is the only right one—it will take total capitulation of the other side for them to "win"—and this outcome is unlikely.

Finally, if both sides are to come to an acceptable agreement and work on good terms afterward, each side must show respect for the other. In line with this, the discussion must not become personal. It cannot end up as one personality against another. The focus must remain on the facts and the issues—not on the characteristics of the individuals on each side. Concentrating on the facts and issues also helps keep both sides working on the problem, and not working against each other.

These guidelines can help resolve a conflict:

- Even if you disagree with the other person's opinions, treat him or her with respect.
- Be convinced that you have enough in common to make communication and a positive result possible.
- Concentrate on the problem. Avoid threats, name-calling, ego involvement, and placing blame for the conflict.
- Report, don't judge. Use descriptive, nonjudgmental terms. Avoid strong, emotion-laden words.
- Be specific. Do not use generalities.
- Discuss the issues most open to change. Avoid those with little or no chance of alteration.
- Discuss one issue at a time. Do not cloud one issue by bringing up something else.

- Stick to the subject. Do not interject items that are not germane to the issue at hand.
- Project a positive image. Show that you are totally confident that things will end positively for both of you.[54]

Although these suggestions cannot prevent or eliminate conflict, or even resolve all conflicts, they can make more conflicts manageable.

Summary

In this chapter we have viewed the communication process as it applies to the working environment. We have seen the impact of nonverbal communication and have seen what managers traditionally expect to receive, especially in unchallenged authority relations. The meaning that can be imparted by messages has been examined. Methods for improving communication and conflict have been discussed.

Knowledge of these areas will make you more aware of them in your own communications and will help you send the message that you intend to. You will understand the communications of others better, and application of the principles outlined in the chapter will improve communications among health workers.

REFERENCES

1. Malandro, B, et al: Nonverbal Communication, ed 2. Random House, New York, 1989, p 13.
2. Mehrabian, A: Silent Messages, ed 2. Wadsworth Publishing, Belmont, Calif., 1981, p 76.
3. Malandro, and Barker, pp 12–14.
4. Ibid, p 30.
5. Sathré-Eldon, FS, et al: Let's Talk, ed 3. Scott, Foresman, Glenview, Ill., 1981, p 60.
6. Molloy, JT: New Dress for Success. Warner Books, New York, 1988, p 1.
7. Malandro, B, Barker, and Barker, p 186.
8. Axtell, RE (ed): Do's and Taboos Around the World, ed 2. John Wiley & Sons, New York, 1990, p 110.
9. Mehrabian, A: Nonverbal Communication. Aldine-Atherton, Chicago, 1972, p 45.
10. Sathré-Eldon, FS, et al, pp 60–61.
11. Fast, J: Subtext: Making Body Language Work in the Workplace. Viking Books, New York, 1991, p 85.
12. Ibid, p 71.
13. Knapp, ML: Essentials of Nonverbal Communication. Holt, Rinehart and Winston, New York, 1980, p 74.
14. Harper, RG, et al: Nonverbal Communication: The State of the Art. John Wiley & Sons, New York, 1978, p 185.
15. Ibid, p 184.
16. Dellinger, S, and Deane, B: Communicating Effectively. Chilton Book Co, Radnor, Penna., 1980, p 72.
17. Sathré-Eldon, FS, et al, p 62.
18. Fast, J, pp 225–228.
19. Sathré-Eldon, et al, p 63.
20. Ruben, BD: Communication and Human Behavior. Macmillan, New York, 1984, p 140.
21. Sathré-Eldon, FS, et al, p 65.
22. Emmert, P, and Donaghy, WC: Human Communication: Elements and Contexts. Addison-Wesley, Reading, Mass., 1981, p 354.
23. Mehrabian, A, Silent Messages, p 84.
24. Vecchio, R: Organizational Behavior, ed 3. Dryden, Fort Worth, TX, 1995, p 549.
25. Dellinger, and Deane, pp 38–39.
26. Sathré-Eldon, et al, p 13.
27. Ibid, p 14.
28. Dellinger, and Deane, p 185.
29. Ibid, p 38.
30. Sathré-Eldon, et al, pp 24–25.
31. Emmert, and Donaghy, p 212.
32. Nelson, D, and Quick, JC: Organizational Behavior. West, St. Paul, Minn., 1994, p 236–37.
33. Briton, N, and Hall, J: Beliefs about female and male nonverbal communication. Sex Roles: A Journal of Research. September 1995, pp 79–90.
34. Tannen, D: You Just Don't Understand. Ballantine Books, New York, 1990, p 43.
35. Ibid, p 62.
36. Gray, J: Men Are from Mars, Women Are from Venus. HarperCollins, New York, 1992, p 17.
37. Ibid, p 16.
38. Ibid, p 29.
39. Ibid, p 60.
40. Tannen, p 43.
41. Ibid, p 49.
42. Gray, J, p 48.
43. Ibid, p 23.
44. Ibid, p 15.
45. Tannen, D: Talking From 9 to 5. William Morrow, New York, 1994, p 13.
46. Gray, J, p 60.
47. Tannen, D, Talking From 9 to 5, p 22.
48. Ibid, p 41.
49. Gray, J, p 29.
50. Ibid, p 117.
51. Ibid, p 60.
52. Emmert, and Donaghy, p 264.
53. Sathré-Eldon, et al, pp 114–116.
54. Betz, BR: Speech Communication and Human Interaction. Scott, Forsman, Glenview, Ill., 1976, p 290.

4 · Economics and Health Care

Objectives

On completion of this chapter, the reader will be able to:

- ☐ Describe the market economic model.
- ☐ Explain the law of supply and demand.
- ☐ Describe the command system.
- ☐ Describe the macroeconomic model.
- ☐ Describe indicative planning.
- ☐ Differentiate between the four economic models.
- ☐ Explain how economics affects the health-care system.
- ☐ Describe the characteristics of the health-care economic environment.
- ☐ List and explain the forces impacting health-care costs.
- ☐ Calculate revenues and expenses for a sample managed care organization.
- ☐ Explain the effects of the law of supply and demand on salary levels.
- ☐ Describe the factors that affect salary structures.
- ☐ List types of compensation other than money.
- ☐ Summarize the effects of economics on the health-care industry.

If you have ever wondered how salaries are determined in the marketplace or what happens to the money that is earned by the delivery of health care, this chapter will help you. In it, we will examine the four general ways in which people organize economically. The most efficient and powerful economy ever devised will be examined, as will the impact of the economy on the health-care industry.

Your role in the economy as an employee will be discussed along with an explanation of employer economics. This explanation will include the ways in which health-care companies may be owned and their characteristics, and the financial decisions that a health-care employer faces. Such a discussion will allow you to understand your position in the economy and the position of employers.

The Four General Economic Models

When economists discuss the various ways that people organize themselves to meet their needs, they talk about economic models. They label them *models* because they represent the ways in which people work together. The models contain theories, many of which are expressed as mathematical formulas. It is beyond the scope of this book to delve deeply into these formulas, which are beyond the needs of most health-care workers. However, it is important to know how economics impacts you as a worker and as a health-care provider.

The ultimate goal of every economy, including the world economy, is to allocate scarce resources.[1] As far as economics is concerned, all resources are scarce. In this context, *scarce* means that there is a finite supply of all resources. The difference between each of the models is in the way each handles the costs of information. The *costs of information* refers to the cost, availability, and need for each item in the economy; that is, the cost of information regarding the supply and demand of each item.

An example should help clarify the meaning of the term cost of information. Let us say that you are going to buy a new car. If a perfect economy is assumed—one where the cost of information is zero—you would pay the lowest price conceivable for your car. However, your access to information is not perfect—it costs something. First of all, how many car dealers will you visit; that is, how many different prices will you get in your search for the lowest? One? Two? Three? Ten? Fifty? The more dealers you go to, the more information (number of prices) you will have, and the greater the chance of your finding the lowest price or negotiating for the lowest price. There is a cost for this information—your time, your money for gas to get to the dealerships, and so on. Shopping costs time and money. This search for data on the price or product you desire is the cost of information. However, this is only one side of the coin.

Producers of goods (cars in the previous example) pay a cost for information also. They need to know how many items to make, which items to make, where to ship them, and what to charge for them. Producers obtain information differently in various economies, some more efficiently, some less so. The more efficiently the information is handled, the better the economy is at allocating scarce resources and the better it is able to meet the needs of its people.

MARKET SYSTEM

The *market* system is one of the two most prevalent economic systems in the world today. It is the cornerstone of the American economy, as it is for most of the world. It is also called the *free market system, free enterprise,* and *capitalism.* The basic philosophy was described by Adam Smith[2,3] in the 1700s, and the most important aspect of a market system is the law of supply and demand.

Although some of Smith's ideas have changed as economies have become more sophisticated, most still apply today. Smith's basic premise was freedom. He said that the economy runs best when people are free to make what they want, free to buy what they want, and free to work where they want.[4] Rather than a government trying to control markets, the markets would be controlled from within by competition. Competition ensures that people get what they want at the lowest prices. For example, if someone is making something that everyone wants and he charges a high price for it, others will see the profits being made and will come out with a version of their own—at a lower price to attract buyers. When people have a choice between the original and the imitator's (at a lower price), the originator will have to lower his price.[5] The process is explained by the law of supply and demand.

The *law of supply and demand* can be used to explain the actions of prices in relation to the amount of goods available. Simply, if the supply of goods increases, the selling price decreases. Conversely, if the supply decreases, the selling price increases. Or, if the demand for something increases, its price will increase; if the demand decreases, the price will decrease.[6] Economists use graphs to depict the supply curve and the demand curve (Fig. 4–1). The intersection of these two lines shows the selling point and the quantity that will be sold in a particular market.

The market system is the best system ever devised to handle the costs of information and allocate resources to meet people's needs. The reason for this success is that there is a feedback loop in the system. As an example, assume that you make two products and offer them for sale simultaneously. You constantly receive new orders for product A. However, you have a 6-month supply of product B in your warehouse gathering dust. You instantly know where to put your resources—into product A. When sales are down and orders are slow, you reduce production of product B. If demand for product B increases later, you can then increase production. If demand for A or B is very high, then others may start to produce items like

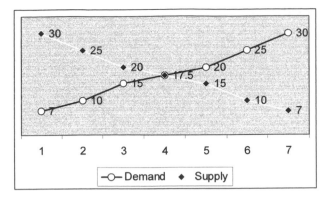

FIGURE 4–1 • As the demand for a product increases (in this case from 1 million to 7 million), the price one can charge for the product increases (from $7 to $30 each). As the supply of a product increases (again, from 1 million to 7 million), the price decreases (from $30 to $7) to entice people to buy. At some point, for every product, the demand for the product at a price most people will pay meets the amount a provider is willing to sell at that price. In this case, if 4 million are made and offered for sale at $17.50 each, they will all be purchased.

them to make some money too. This constant return of sales information allows producers to know what products and services to make—make what sells; charge what the market will bear—and which to stop making.

This same system works in providing health-care services and in allocating salaries of health-care professionals.

COMMAND SYSTEM

The *command system* is another of the basic ways in which an economy can be organized. The system is based on a hierarchy, or chain, of command. The top person (or people) passes orders to the next lowest level, then to the next, and the next, and so on (Fig. 4–2). This system is also called central planning, and it is the basis for dictatorships and socialist systems. Proponents believe that its advantages include control and uniformity. As a basis for an entire economy, the system has generally failed, as seen by the fall of the USSR's command system and the subsequent introduction of capitalism in formerly socialist countries of Europe and in Russia.[7]

One of the major problems with the command system as a basis for an economy is that it does not handle the costs of information well. Primarily, the quantity, type, and price of goods are planned (that is, guessed at) by the central planning commission. The natural feedback loop of the market system and freedom to choose and produce many products is not present. You can get an idea of how difficult the task is from the following example:

Let us assume that you are going to build a hospital and health-care offices in a central planning country. To do so, you must list all the components that go into the hospital on the left side of a matrix (Table 4–1). This task may seem challenging, but is easy. Then list how much of each item is needed in the box to the right of each item—another challenge, but manageable.

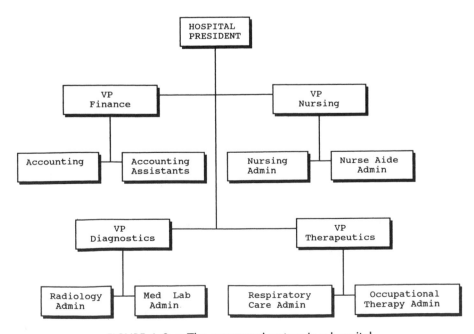

FIGURE 4–2 • The command system in a hospital.

TABLE 4–1 • COMPONENTS OF A HOSPITAL

	Hospital	Trucks	Equipment	Homes	Schools
Steel					
Glass					
Concrete					
Bricks					
Mortar					
Roofing					
Electrical					
Furnaces					
Air conditioners					
Beds					
Doors					
Elevators					
People					

Next, in the other columns, list the amount of materials needed for the people that will build this hospital and offices. Add things like food, shelter, and clothing that are not in the list of hospital items that these people need. Then, list the materials needed for the people and plants to produce these items. For instance, steel is needed for the buildings, medical equipment, housing for the workers, and the workers' tools. Steel must also be planned for and produced for the factories that make the components of the hospital, the vehicles that bring the components to the work site, the factories to make the trucks, and the factories to make the steel for the trucks and buildings. Steel will also be needed for the housing for the workers making the steel for the factories that will make the steel for the tools that will build the other steel into a hospital! And steel is just one item for one type of building. We won't even mention the schools needed to educate all the people involved in this one part of the process (and housing and cars for the teachers, and so on). Even using the largest computers, it is not possible to successfully manage an entire economy in this manner. It is not surprising then that industrial socialist economies failed miserably.

There are applications for the command system in every economy, however. Command systems do function if they are significantly smaller than those required to run an entire country. Almost every organization, including the military and the government, uses the command system in the form of the chain of command. For businesses, the command system provides an effective method of maintaining control, standards, and uniform outputs (products and services). However, the empha-

sis on downward communication is a problem in governments and business command systems.

MACROECONOMIC MODEL

The *macroeconomic model* is popular, but it is not used alone. It is used with another method like the market system. As the name implies, it is used to measure and manipulate large segments of the economy. The following are some of these segments:

- Unemployment
- Inflation
- Money supply
- Interest rates
- Gross domestic product

Some of these segments may be familiar because they are frequently reported in the news.

In using macroeconomics, the government attempts to influence economic conditions to avoid depressions and times of high inflation. Some had felt that these business cycles were a fact of life, and the best that could be done was to try to predict when they would occur. However, the Great Depression of the 1930s was so deep that a solution was desperately sought.

Enter John Maynard Keynes. Keynes was British, and he had developed a mathematical model to explain the workings of a market economy. The detailed equations are complex, but the basic equation is, like many brilliant discoveries, quite simple. Keynes started looking at the source of everyone's income. He wanted to explain where the money comes from that makes up everyone's paycheck. He came up with three sources. Some paychecks come from what others spend on consumer goods, C. Other incomes result from business investment spending for new factories and equipment, I. The rest comes from people working for the government, G. Then he looked at where the money in the paychecks went. Much of it went to buy consumer goods, C. The government received some as taxes, T, and if anything was left over, people saved it, S. He then put this all together in one equation, using, y, to represent incomes (having used I for business investment spending). Thus, the entire economy can be simply represented by:

$$C + I + G = y = C + S + T$$

Consuming + business investment + government spending
= incomes = consuming + savings + taxes

and

$$C = C$$

Consuming (consumer spending) = consuming (consumer spending)

$$G = T$$

Government spending = taxes

$$I = S$$

Business investment = savings

Simple algebra tells you that $C = C$. We also know that government spending comes from taxes, so that $G = T$. This means that $I = S$, or business gets money for investment spending by borrowing from the bank the money everyone else saves. The important part is that if one side of the equation decreases, then y decreases; and then the other side must decrease. If $C + I + G$ decreases, y decreases, and $C + S + T$ decreases; but that causes $C + I + G$ to decrease again, and y decreases again, and $C + S + T$ decreases again. This declining spiral continues until the economy is ruined—or until someone starts increasing spending. However, the only entity that can spend more than it takes in is the government. In the 1930s Keynes convinced the U.S. government to do just that. The spiral then began to work in reverse. So as the G in $C + I + G$ increased, y increased, and people had more to spend. Thus $C + S + T$ increased, and the economy recovered.[8]

Since Keynes's time, the government has used macroeconomics to try to keep the economy growing but at a pace that does not cause high inflation nor high unemployment. This is no small task owing in part to the complexity of the economy and in part to the fact that inflation and unemployment

work in opposition. As unemployment goes up, inflation is supposed to go down. Actually, the system worked rather well until the mid-1960s. This was a time when G, government spending, should have decreased to avoid inflation. However, the Vietnam War was going on, and President Johnson had his Great Society social programs passed through Congress, and the war and the social programs cost a large amount of money. Johnson did not reduce spending on either issue, and the elected officials in Congress did not reduce spending either.

Keynesian economics did not have a ready solution for this problem. In addition, since that time, artificially high oil prices have often upset the system. Today, macroeconomics is still widely used, but it is not a cure-all for the economy. Part of the problem is the Keynesian economics was developed to work with the economy of one country. Presently the economies of most of the industrialized countries and many of the industrializing countries are highly interrelated. Keynesian economics was not designed to account for the vast amounts of direct investment and trade of many nations. Unfortunately, no one else has devised a system that can take enough of the facets of today's economies into account.

INDICATIVE PLANNING

Indicative planning is the fourth economic model, and it is the system used by Japan, in conjunction with a market system. This is a method of planning that allows different producers to meet with the government to set policies for the good of the people. It is dissimilar to central planning, which has an imperative plan. In the indicative planning system, as its name implies, companies give the government an indication of what they plan to do.[9]

As an example, assume that five producers meet with the government agency that studies their segment of the economy. The government would say, "250,000 of your products are needed this year. How many do each of you intend to make?" Each producer would write down a number and give it to the government representative. Let us say that each intends to make 100,000. The total, 500,000, would be announced. The government person would say, "If you all produce this number, you will not sell what you make. With this new information, give me a new estimate." Now Producer A still says 100,000, and the rest say 50,000 each. The new total of 300,000 is announced, and they go around again. This continues until the group agrees to 250,000. No individual was forced to change. In fact, Producer A stayed at 100,000 throughout (Fig. 4–3). In the end, they are all free to do what they

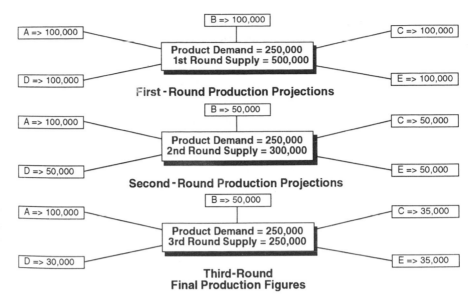

FIGURE 4–3 • Indicative planning in action. Initially these five producers would have made twice as much product as is needed by consumers. With governmental assistance, production figures are voluntarily changed to match demand.

want. However, they know that if they stick to their indications, they will sell all they make.

This method is very different from the American system. In fact, following the scenario above, Americans would have been jailed for conspiracy in restraint of trade (that is, trying to form a trust or monopoly). This system works in Japan because the Japanese culture is group or community oriented, rather than individualistic as in Western cultures. However, indicative planning was used in America to put the first man on the moon. The difference there was that virtually everyone in the country agreed to the common goal that America would be the first to land on the moon, and the government and private industry worked together to carry out the will of the people for the lowest cost possible.

Health-care Economics

Health-care facilities are affected by, and must survive in, our economic system. Because one of the cornerstones of our economy is competition, we will examine this aspect of our system first.

In a typical market, people produce goods or provide services and advertise them along with their prices. Consumers then shop and compare and make a purchase based on paying what they consider to be a fair price for the good or service. It is also common to have different levels of price, quality, and features available. How might this system work in health care?

Let us say that you need rotator cuff surgery. You might get the Sunday papers to see who was offering a sale on the surgery this week. After finding some possibilities, you could go see a few surgeons

and talk about price. Maybe one promises 30 stitches instead of 20 for a nicer scar. You might talk another into including a free bunionectomy. A third might have a package with free physical therapy services; with the others such service would be extra or you would have to find your own. The deluxe package might come prearranged with front-door pickup, anesthesiology, medical imaging, laboratory work, nursing care, and at-home physical therapy—for a deluxe price, of course. Maybe some surgeons offer a warranty—2 years or 2000 abductions or circumductions, whichever comes first. Although this may seem quite amusing, it is basically the way the rest of our economy works.

The way competition is handled is one of the ways health care in the United States differs from the rest of the economy. There is very little, if any, open competition. By *open competition,* I mean the kind depicted above—competition based on price with various levels of service available to suit your pocketbook. In fact, it is only recently that medical advertising of any kind has been allowed. However, there is competition.

As the number of health facilities increases, price should decrease as each facility tries to maintain or increase the number of patients it has. The picture is complicated because the competition is almost covert. State and local governments generally restrict the number of health-care facilities, especially hospitals, in a given area. Before enlarging or building new facilities, administrators are required to prove that sufficient unmet demand exists for more services, and they typically must obtain a certificate of need. The competition then often occurs in the hearing rooms, not in the marketplace. Any restriction of supply (such as this) increases prices. Restricting the number of health-care providers by limiting admissions to training programs or by requiring providers to obtain a license (after meeting certain criteria) also leads to higher prices.

Not having full, open competition leads to higher costs of medicine. This is not the entire story, however. First, notice that I said "higher," not "high." The lack of competition *leads to* higher prices, which is much different from saying it "causes" high prices. Second, controlling the number of health-care workers by requiring them to meet standards may increase costs, but the alternative of insufficiently trained workers would be far worse. Third, having open competition would not guarantee low prices—there is a certain standard of care demanded by Americans that all facilities would have to provide to be successful, and that care is costly.

Americans expect a very high level of health care.[10] This is one reason why the system is one of the best in the world. However, as mentioned, it is also very expensive. In every other area of the marketplace, you can find goods and services at various prices with quality that usually matches. However, that is not true in health care. For the most part, we expect the best equipment and the highest standards of care at every facility. People will even sue if they think they received less than the best. Although this analogy has been used before, it still applies: It is as if everyone wants Cadillac care; no one is willing to settle for bare-essentials, Hyundai or Kia care. This means that every health-care facility must have a full range of basic services available. And this basic level is relatively high when compared to other areas in the economy. Compare merchandise and service at a discount clothing store and a custom men's or women's clothier. We expect health facilities to be closer to the high end of the spectrum than the low end. These expectations have an important effect on competition.

The demand for high-level care exerts an upward pressure on prices.[11] If twice as many facilities were introduced into an area, prices should decrease. In health care, prices would probably *increase*. Why? Because each facility would be expected to have basically a full range of services. At a deep discount store you might be willing to bag your own groceries; can you imagine a deep discount medical facility where you stitch your own incision, mix your own prescription, do your own EKG? Having twice as many services available to the same number of clients would be wasteful. For example, let us say that a particular city has medical needs requiring one 400-bed hospital with all the trimmings. Should the prices not be the same or less if there were two 200-bed facilities? Probably not. Each would be expected to be able to provide essentially the same services in the same amount of time. Some resources would sit idle or be underutilized. The costs for the duplication of effort that would exist would be borne by the patients. Thus the net result could be higher prices because there would be no savings from economies of scale (savings from one magnetic resonance imaging [MRI] scanner for 12 hours a day at one 400-bed hospital as opposed to two scanners each used for 6 hours a day at the two 200-bed hospitals).

Essentially everyone wants the highest level of care available. However, what people want and what they get are often two entirely different things. Why isn't there a limit on the amount of care a person can get? Why are seemingly needless (and expensive) tests performed? There are two main reasons: one ethical, the other legal. Ethically, it is extremely difficult to limit health care. Very few people are willing to tell someone that they can't have a test or a therapy because it will not be paid for. The basic philosophy of health care is to do everything possible for every patient. Limiting health care requires God-like decisions that would appear extremely cold or cruel if made on some logical basis, or discriminatory if made in some other way. There are also legal reasons not to limit health care.

In the case of a legal dispute over a patient's care, saying that there were insufficient funds to pay for an examination or treatment would not be much of a defense in many courts. It is almost a requirement that all possibilities be exhausted until the problem is found or until there is documentation that none was found. To do less is to risk a lawsuit and a large settlement on behalf of the patient if it later turns out that the patient did have a problem. Although limited competition and third-party payers (insurance companies, governments, and so on) try to hold down costs, the courts and people's expectations often force them up.

There are still factors that affect health-care economics including the technology, the people involved, and the supply of employees. Part of the upward trend in health-care costs is directly attributable to the level of technology involved. In the last 25 years medicine has moved into high-technology areas. From medical imaging to intensive care to transplant technology, expensive, computerized equipment can be seen almost everywhere. Although technology has been of benefit to the patients, it is still very expensive. As one example, an MRI scanner and installation can cost millions of dollars. Adding to the problem, as mentioned previously, is that once one facility has a certain kind of equipment, others are almost compelled to obtain it, or lose their clientele. Although some facilities have attempted to share equipment, this practice has not been successful nor widely applied.

Although more and more high-technology equipment is being employed, for the most part it has not replaced or decreased the need for health-care workers. And health care is a labor-intensive industry. Capital-intensive industries, those that are automated, have significant initial costs, but over time are much more economical. Labor-intensive industries are continuously expensive. To date, there have been few areas in health care, other than laboratory testing, that have been successfully automated.

Labor-intensive industries are not only expensive, but they are subject to fluctuations in the supply of workers. When there is a decrease in the number of workers because fewer people are attracted to the field or there is a general lack of workers (as in a "baby-bust"), the costs of labor generally increase. You might think that if employers can't find workers, they can at least save the cost of their salaries. However, the few savings are usually more than offset by increases needed in recruitment, lost productivity, overtime pay, and salaries for the workers that are available.

MANAGED CARE

Beginning in the 1960s and 1970s, health-care costs began to increase dramatically.[12] The introduction of Medicare and Medicaid is often mentioned as the cause, but malpractice insurance premiums, high patient expectations, defensive medicine, increasingly expensive medical equipment, more expensive drugs, and medical insurance in general all contributed.[13] High patient expectations, more expensive malpractice insurance, and defensive medicine are all related. As mentioned earlier in this chapter, most people in the United States have come to expect the best health care possible. Advances in medicine also raised expectations to the point that many people who became ill expected the medical community to be able to cure them rather quickly. When a cure failed, more and more people sued for damages. It seems that many people expected every health-care provider to know all and be able to cure all. Medicine began to be perceived to be all science and not at all art. If recovery from a disease was not complete, many believed that somone made a mistake and had to be made to pay for the mistake. Juries would often enough be sympathetic to the patient and award huge sums of money. These sums were paid by insurance companies who then had to increase the price for insurance policies (the premiums). Health-care providers had to then increase fees to cover the insurance premiums, and, to avoid missing any conditions, physicians started ordering many more tests to

"rule out" even the remotest possibility, a practice referred to as *defensive medicine*. The general rule at the time was to order a procedure not because a condition was suspected, but to obtain proof that *no* condition was present at the time.

As if these pressures on health-care costs were not enough, expensive technologies were being introduced at about the same time. Advances in medications also contributed to the problem. It wasn't that the cost of making the medicines had really increased, it was the many years needed to find new medicines and the extensive tests required before the medications could be used. The extensive testing did help protect patients to a very large degree (as when thalidomide, a drug which can cause massive birth defects was kept off the U.S. markets) but it also added to cost increases. Medical insurance in general also increased the costs by not providing health-care providers or patients with any reason to hold costs down. This third-party payer system, expanded by Medicare and Medicaid, removed a vital link from our economic system. Imagine how life would be today if someone else paid for your food and never asked questions; they paid for whatever you bought. Without having to personally pay, many people would select the best food and more of it. That is what health care was like in the '60s and '70s. Your physician could order, and you could have, almost any procedure desired, and someone else paid for it. With all of these factors added together, health-care spending was out of control.[14]

To try to control the increasing costs of health care, the U.S. Congress pushed to establish some type of supervision of the number and types of procedures being ordered. Rather than the fee-for-service system (a procedure is performed, a fee charged, and the fee paid, with virtually no questions asked) a system was devised where one fee would be paid each year and all of a person's medical needs would be covered. This began the era of managed care.

Managed care refers to providing health-care services by a limited number of health-care professionals for a fixed prepaid fee.[15] That fixed fee is called a *capitated payment*.[16] A managed care system also has the responsibility of providing quality health care that is cost effective. With the support of government and business, the concept of managed care progressed with the initial development of Medicare, Medicaid, and health maintenance organizations (HMOs), and the later development of preferred provider organizations (PPOs) and point of service (POS) plans. No matter what the form of the managed care organization (MCO), all of them in some way restrict the access their members have to health care.[17] Members may be restricted in their access to specialists (they may need a primary care physician's approval first), or they may have to select a physician or hospital from a list of those affiliated or approved by the MCO, or the type of approved treatments or medications may be limited. Various MCOs trade costs for freedom of choice. Plans that allow covered members more freedom to choose their health-care provider cost more money; lower costs mean less freedom to choose.

Management of care (and costs) in many MCOs is essentially handled by the primary care physician (PCP). The PCP acts as a regulator by first determining whether or not a patient needs to see a specialist or whether an outpatient procedure can be performed rather than a more expensive inpatient procedure. Although it may seem more costly to require possibly two doctor visits (the PCP and then a specialist), costs are supposed to be lower because only contract specialists are used. Other ways costs are minimized in MCOs include requiring patients to have an office visit rather than go to an emergency department (the ED provides faster treatment but is much more expensive), restricting access to newer (and typically more expensive) drugs, and employing utilization review (UR). Utilization review is a means of examining decisions and comparing the care provided to guidelines for the person's condition. Utilization review may determine that a treatment or procedure was so far outside of the guidelines that payment is refused.[18]

HMOs were the first MCOs to attempt to oversee runaway health-care costs. HMOs were to emphasize preventative medicine. Rather than just treat people once they became ill, HMOs would try to keep people from becoming ill in the first place.[19] They received a fixed annual fee for each member, which was also designed to manage costs. As a result, there was no incentive to order unneeded tests because there would be no extra money beyond the annual fee. If an HMO spent less money than the annual fee received, it was allowed to keep the money. If it spent more that the annual fee, it would have to absorb the cost itself. The problem all HMOs (and really all MCOs) face is that if some patients use more money than allowed, then it must be hoped that the extra can be saved on other patients who use less. Because these organizations do not know what expenses or savings are in the future, there is considerable pressure to limit the spending on each and every patient.[20] It is for this reason that people have complained most about managed care in general and specifically about HMOs for sometimes denying emergency department care or denying new, less tested (and costly) treatments.

There are four main types of HMOs—staff, group,

IPA, and network.[21] In staff HMOs, the health-care providers are employees of the HMO, and they provide care only for HMO members. In group HMOs, the care is provided not by employees of the HMO but by a separate group of physicians. A contract binds the physician organization to the HMO, and the physician group agrees to treat only members of the HMO. In IPA HMOs, there are contracts between the HMO and individual physicians. The individual physicians use their own offices to treat HMO patients, and they also treat non-HMO patients. Network HMOs are the fourth main type of HMO. These are similar to IPA HMOs except that instead of contracts with individual physicians, the HMO has contracts with a number of large physician groups. Those groups treat HMO patients as well as non-HMO patients.

Even with HMOs, Medicare, and Medicaid costs for health care in the 1980s were still not under control. Medicare then tried to decrease costs by applying a formula to determine how much would be paid for every type of disease and condition. The system of various diseases and conditions was termed Diagnosis Related Groups, or DRGs. Before DRGs, Medicare would just pay whatever it was billed. The DRG system determined the average cost for an illness and paid that amount. If your health-care provider's costs were lower, Medicare kept the extra money; if the costs were greater, then the health-care provider had to hope the loss could be made up from situations where the costs were lower.[22] This was a large incentive to, for example, get a patient in and out of the hospital in 2 days rather than 10. DRGs addressed hospital costs only, however.

To handle physician costs, a counterpart to DRGs was created. Here, a physician voluntarily agreed to accept only the amount Medicare "assigned." Under the assignment system, patients paid some of the costs and physicians could still charge whatever they wanted, but Medicare only paid the assigned amount. This was supposed to provide patients with the motivation to see only physicians accepting assignments because the patient would pay less. Patients paid 20 percent of the assignment, but would have to pay whatever the difference was between the assignment and what a nonparticipating physician felt like charging.[23]

In 1992 a further effort was made to restrain physician fees through the Resource-based Relative Value System (RBRVS). Prior to the RBRVS doctors received more money for performing a physical task than they received for performing a cognitive (thinking) task. RBRVS uses units of effort for both performance and knowledge tasks.[24] The RBRVS was intended to move money from

 Building Comprehension Exercise begins on following page

BUILDING COMPREHENSION EXERCISE 4–1

Operating a Managed-care Organization (MCO)

In this exercise you will see what it is like to operate a managed care organization. In your MCO you have 67,000 members, and you charged $11,000 for each to cover costs for 1 year. Your task is to calculate costs for each quarter, report on the status of your funds, and make an important decision after the 3rd quarter. (Note: If your calculator does not handle hundreds of millions [9 digits], you may leave off the last 3 digits and calculate everything in thousands of dollars. So 737,000,000 becomes 737,000 thousands [737 million is then 737 thousand thousands].) Items in boldface type are used elsewhere in the exercise.

First, how much money do you have to work with?

67,000 × $11,000 = _____

Subtract administrative costs to run the MCO.

_____ − $66,000,000

What is left to pay all of the member medical claims for the year?

Yearly Budget = _____

How much can you spend on all of the member medical claims for each quarter?

_____ / 4 = _____

Yearly Budget **Quarterly**
divided by **4** **Budget**

How much can you spend on each member each quarter?

_____ / 67,000 = _____

Quarterly Budget divided by 67,000

Now we need to calculate the MCO's financial condition quarter by quarter.

1st Quarter

Enter your Quarterly Budget amount on this line. _____

Claims for the 1st Quarter. (Subtract from Quarterly Budget.) − $107, 669,000

This is the 1st Quarter Budget Variance. Is it positive or negative? _____

What are your Cash Reserves? Enter Yearly Budget figure here. _____

Subtract 1st Quarter Claims. − $107, 669,000

Cash Reserves after the 1st Quarter = _____

Exercise continues on following page ❂ ❂ ❂

2nd Quarter

Enter your Quarterly Budget amount on this line.   _____

Claims for the 2nd Quarter. (Subtract from Quarterly Budget.)   − $226,393,000

This is the 2nd Quarter Budget Variance. Is it positive or negative?   _____

What are your Cash Reserves?

Enter Cash Reserves after the 1st Quarter here.   _____

Subtract 2nd Quarter Claims.   − $226,393,000

Cash Reserves after the 2nd Quarter =   _____

3rd Quarter

Enter your Quarterly Budget amount on this line.   _____

Claims for the 3rd Quarter. (Subtract from Quarterly Budget.)   − $212,189,000

This is the 3rd Quarter Budget Variance. Is it positive or negative?   _____

What are your Cash Reserves?

Enter Cash Reserves after the 2nd Quarter here.   _____

Subtract 2nd Quarter Claims.   − $212,189,000

Cash Reserves after the 3rd Quarter =   _____

Let's see how things are going.

Compare your Cash Reserves after the 3rd Quarter
to the Quarterly Budget.   _____

Subtract the Quarterly Budget from 3rd Quarter Reserves.   _____

If the result is a positive number the MCO is doing well. If the result is a negative number the MCO is not doing well.

4th Quarter

Calculate how much money is left to spend per MCO member.

Enter the Cash Reserves after the 3rd Quarter here.   _____

Divide this by the number of members.   / 67,000

The result is how much is left for each member.   _____

Exercise continues on following page ❧ ❧ ❧

This is also the influenza season. There is a new drug on the market, Outfluenza, which is very effective in minimizing the duration and severity of the flu. However, it must be taken within 8 hours of the first symptoms and then again 8 and 16 hours after the first dose. This means that members need Outfluenza in their homes just in case they think they are starting to get sick. This costs $49 per member for a total of $3,283,000. Do you supply Outfluenza to all MCO members or not?

IF YOU SAID "**YES**" AND BOUGHT ALL MEMBERS OUTFLUENZA, USE THESE NUMBERS:

4th Quarter

Enter your Quarterly Budget amount on this line.   _____

Subtract the cost of Outfluenza.   − $3,283,000

Remaining 4th Quarter Budget.   _____

Claims for the 4th quarter. (Subtract from remaining Quarterly Budget.)   − $139,963,000

This is the 4th Quarter Budget Variance. Is it positive or negative?   _____

What are your Cash Reserves?

Enter Cash Reserves after the 3rd Quarter here.   _____

Subtract the cost of Outfluenza.   − $3,283,000

Remaining Cash Reserves.   _____

Subtract 4th Quarter Claims.   − $139,963,000

Cash Reserves FOR THE YEAR =   _____

If the Cash Reserves For The Year are positive, you made a profit. If the Cash Reserves For The Year are negative, you lost money.

IF YOU SAID "**NO**" AND DID NOT BUY ALL MEMBERS OUTFLUENZA, USE THESE NUMBERS:

4th Quarter

Enter your Quarterly Budget amount on this line.   _____

Claims for the 4th Quarter. (Subtract from Quarterly Budget.)   − $249,441,000

This is the 4th Quarter Budget Variance. Is it positive or negative?   _____

What are your Cash Reserves?

Enter Cash Reserves after the 3rd Quarter here.   _____

Subtract 4th Quarter Claims.   − $249,441,000

Cash Reserves FOR THE YEAR =   _____

Exercise continues on following page ❧❧❧

If the Cash Reserves For The Year are positive, you made a profit. If the Cash Reserves For The Year are negative, you lost money.

How did you do? What should you do differently next year? Examine the Quarterly Budget Variances. Which quarters or conditions hurt most (i.e., the Variance was negative)?

_____

_____

_____

_____

Figure the 4th Quarter with and without buying Outfluenza. In this case, does buying Outfluenza cost more money, or was it actually cheaper to let people get sick and just treat them afterwards? What is the best financial decision? What is the correct ethical decision?

_____

_____

_____

_____

What would you have done if it turned out to be cheaper to let people get the flu rather than buy the Outfluenza?

_____

_____

_____

_____

End of exercise. Text continues on following page.
Answers to Exercise 4–1 are in the Appendix at the end of this chapter.

more expensive specialist physicians to less costly general practitioners. So far, the effect has been less than hoped for.

At about this same time other variations of MCOs became increasingly noticeable. PPOs consist of networks of hospitals, doctors, and other health-care providers who treat patients for a negotiated fee. PPOs are typically offered as an option (or rider) to a traditional health insurance plan. PPOs are not involved in making decisions on treatment, and they assume no financial risk. HMOs do both. Essentially, PPOs negotiate reduced fees from a very wide range of health-care providers, mostly for insurance companies and employers who are self-insured. PPO members typically have a great degree of freedom of choice in selecting health-care providers from within the PPO network.[25] Another variation of an MCO is the POS plan. POS plans have a network of approved health-care providers, but they give members even greater freedom by allowing them to also select providers from outside the network. As mentioned before, with virtually all MCOs this increased freedom comes with an increased cost, and the POS is not an exception.[26]

Although some people have argued against managed care as a form of rationing health care and as simply additional layers of costly bureaucracy, an economic argument in favor of managed care can be made. Proponents of managed care can claim that is has forced a better allocation of scarce medical resources and it has forced more standard care.[27] It has reduced the incentive or temptation to order vast batteries of tests because managed care will not simply pay whatever is charged. Also, by approving and reviewing care according to guidelines, more consistency has been introduced into the system and controlling costs has forced a reduction in waste.

ADDITIONAL FACTORS

Two additional factors that tend to increase health costs include the aging population and the ability to sustain life. Older people require more health care than younger people do. Obviously this increases health-care costs. Because many older people are retired, their health-care expenses are added to other costs that third-party payers (insurance and Medicare) must pay. And, medical technology is now capable of sustaining a body almost indefinitely. When this technology is used, it increases cost not only in the short term from its immediate use but also in the long term because it may keep someone alive who would otherwise have died (and efforts to end this care when recovery is hopeless are very controversial).

In summation, this section has demonstrated that:

- The health-care market is significantly different from other markets in the economy.
- In health care, some elements of the market system exist, and competition is a modified version from that seen in other markets.
- The high level of care demanded by the public exerts an upward pressure on health costs.
- The number of malpractice cases and the high awards to patients encourage defensive medicine in which tests are performed almost as much to provide documentation in case of a lawsuit as to diagnose a disease. Such defensive medicine increases health costs.
- Increasing use of high-technology equipment pushes costs higher.
- The fact that health care is a labor-intensive industry increases costs.
- An aging population and the ability to sustain life with the use of technology also tend to increase costs.

Employee Economics

COMPENSATION

Money

Money is not the only reason people work, but it is usually high on most people's lists. Of course, few people actually want money for its own sake. What they really want are the things that money can buy. Money just happens to be a much more convenient way to handle transactions. It would be impossible to run a modern society on a barter system, for example. This section will examine the method that determines how much money a person receives for working.

The basic determinant of salary levels is the law of supply and demand.[28] As mentioned earlier, if the supply of something decreases or if the demand for it increases, its price will rise. Salaries are the price employers are willing to pay for the labor or services of employees. If, for example, there had been a supply of 100 workers of a certain type and suddenly 25 of them left the area, salary levels would increase. They would have to increase in order for employers to attract workers from other employers in the area and to induce workers from other areas to move. On the other hand, if instead of 25 employees leaving, 25 moved into the area, salaries would stay the same or fall. Employers would not have to pay more because there would be additional people to fill the positions—people just waiting for an opening. A number of questions typically accompany this explanation:

1. How are salaries initially established?
2. Why don't they fluctuate more?
3. Why are some workers doing the same job as others who are paid more?

The law of supply and demand works to set the salaries not only for particular classes of workers but for all workers. Salaries are set within professions by the number available in a certain geographic area. They are also set in relation to other professions in the area. Let us examine the cases of a maintenance worker who replaces light bulbs, a maintenance worker one who cleans floors, and a surgeon. The surgeon receives the highest salary. It is not as easy to tell which maintenance worker receives more money. But what is more important here is why the surgeon receives more. The answer does not lie in which position is more valuable. The surgeon needs the maintenance people, for surgery cannot be performed with dirty floors and no lights. However, the surgeon could do the maintenance jobs, but not vice versa. And the surgeon's job requires more education, more rare skills and abilities, and more experience. The surgeon is not paid based on these facts though. Instead, these requirements limit the number of people who can become surgeons. Because the supply of surgeons is limited, surgeons receive a certain salary. Because there are many more people who could change light bulbs and wash floors, these people receive less money than the surgeon.

There is another aspect of the law of supply and demand that applies to wages. If there is an increase in demand or a decrease in the supply of a certain group of workers, then salaries for that group will eventually rise.[29] However, this higher wage makes the work look more appealing to others, who will then enter the workforce, increasing the supply of that group of workers and decreasing the demand. This increase in supply will cause salaries to fall. However, if this increase in demand is fulfilled by an increase in supply in a short amount of time, salaries may not change at all. The longer it takes for people to prepare for a profession, the greater the pressure on salaries to rise (because the demand will remain unfilled longer).[30]

The fact that the time between an increase in demand being met by an increase in supply is not always long enough to increase salaries helps to explain why salaries do not fluctuate more widely or more rapidly. There are other reasons too. First, employers have salary structures; that is, a system for employee compensation.[31] Employers are frequently reluctant to change one part of this structure because of ramifications to other parts. For example, a friend of mine recently told me about a hospital that was experiencing a shortage of workers in department A and a slight surplus in department B. To alleviate the problem, the salary for new employees in department A was paid for by reducing the wages of the current workers in department B. It is not hard to imagine how the workers in department B felt about this. Not only were relations between the two departments increasingly strained, but the attitudes of department B workers toward the employer declined greatly.

A second reason that salaries do not fluctuate like prices for other commodities is that it takes a relatively long time to establish that there is a shortage or excess of workers. Also, it usually takes a shortage of more than one or two workers before an employer decides to change salaries. Finally, salaries do not decrease rapidly for the opposite reasons they do not increase rapidly, and especially because of the effect on current employees. Even though an employer might be able to save a few cents by lowering salaries because demand is down, it does not mean he or she will do it. The damaging effects to the current employees often far outweigh the amounts that could be saved.

The third commonly asked question about salaries concerns the various salary levels within a job class.[32–35] It is not unusual to see variations for the following reasons (but usually not all are seen in the same job class):

- Level of education
- Amount of experience
- Employee skills
- Employee abilities
- Seniority
- Responsibility
- Time of day worked
- Geographic location
- Local costs
- Financial condition of the firm
- Quantity of work
- Quality of work

Many of these are beyond the law of supply and demand as it applies to salaries; in fact, they are part of the inducements employers use to lure and retain workers. But, because they do impact salaries and can influence an employee's decision to work for an employer, they will be examined here.

Level of education affects supply by filtering out those who cannot reach a particular level. It may also be used to justify paying one employee in a certain job class more than another who does not have the degree. However, in some jobs, the skills an employee possesses may be more important than or equally as important as the degree.

Generally, employees with more experience at a particular job are paid more to perform that job than workers new to the field. The belief is that there has been learning to accompany the experience, thus enabling the worker to perform at a higher level or with fewer errors.

Employees with additional skills are sometimes paid extra for them. They may receive the higher wage because they can operate an additional or special piece of equipment or because they can perform procedures that others cannot.

Employees with extra abilities may be compensated at a higher rate. They may possess the same skills as other employees; however, if they have the ability to speak another language or interpret sign language, they may be compensated for handling all of the situations where these are needed.

Seniority is a common method for differentiating pay. Basically the only difference between seniority and experience is that experience is time spent with employers, whereas seniority is time spent with the same employer. This does not mean that the two are compensated equally. Employers often value the time spent with their company more than that spent with others.

Sometimes employees receive additional compensation for taking on added responsibility. An employee may agree to take inventory or perform scheduling in return for an increase in pay.

Another common factor by which salaries within a job class are differentiated is the time of day worked. This is also known as a shift differential. Employees working evening shifts usually receive more money than those on day shifts; and night shifts pay more than evening shifts. People working weekends and holidays are often paid at a higher rate, too.

Geographic location can affect pay rates too. For example, to attract workers from the suburbs, inner-city employers may have to pay more to offset the time and cost of the additional travel. This may also work in reverse. Beyond local areas there can be wide fluctuation because of geography. Remoteness and climate are two other factors employers may have to take into account when devising salary structures.

Local costs also affect remuneration. A location may be desirable geographically, allowing for lower salaries, but if local costs are high, salaries may have to rise also. Hawaii is a good example.

The near-perfect climate would tend to attract many people, increasing supply and decreasing salaries. But the cost of living is high, so salaries are pressed higher so that people can afford to live there.

It should be obvious that the financial condition of the firm can impact salaries. The firm cannot pay out what it does not have. It is amazing, however, how many workers do not see the connection. Some do not see that if they are not productive, not only is the company hurt, but so are the workers. There can be no raise without some profit, and there can be no jobs without some income.

Quantity of work can also account for variations in earnings. Some people are paid per unit of work rather than by the hour or by an annual salary. This is also known as being paid a piece rate. In the health fields there are people who are paid per patient or client. Another way in which quantity affects pay is when employers pay a higher hourly or salary rate because the employees are expected to do more than at comparable firms.

Finally, quality of work can also be a base for differences in emolument. People producing higher-quality work or that with a lower repeat or reject rate may be paid at a higher rate.

Fringe Benefits

Employers frequently offer compensation other than money to their employees, especially to full-time employees.[36-38] These fringe benefits are quite costly but have come to be expected by most workers. Most are self-explanatory. They include:

- Vacations
- Holidays
- Sick leave
- Health insurance
- Dental insurance
- Life insurance
- Insurance for dependents
- Disability insurance
- Retirement programs
- Tuition reimbursement
- Continuing education opportunities
- Employee assistance programs
- Day care
- Leaves of absence
- Flexible work schedules

Employee assistance programs may need a brief explanation. These are programs frequently run by

BUILDING COMPREHENSION EXERCISE 4–2

Rating Your Benefits

Rate the importance of each of these employer-provided benefits to you today (VI=Very Important, I=Important, and NI=Not Important). Then rank those you rated as Very Important and Important, with 1 being the most important. Finally, repeat the procedure evaluating the importance of these benefits to you as you imagine they will be 15 years from now.

Current Evaluation   **Future Evalua**

VI I NI Rank   VI I NI Rank

___ ___ ___ ___   Vacations   ___ ___ ___ ___

___ ___ ___ ___   Holidays   ___ ___ ___ ___

___ ___ ___ ___   Sick leave   ___ ___ ___ ___

___ ___ ___ ___   Health insurance   ___ ___ ___ ___

___ ___ ___ ___   Dental insurance   ___ ___ ___ ___

___ ___ ___ ___   Life insurance   ___ ___ ___ ___

___ ___ ___ ___   Insurance for dependents   ___ ___ ___ ___

___ ___ ___ ___   Disability insurance   ___ ___ ___ ___

___ ___ ___ ___   Retirement programs   ___ ___ ___ ___

___ ___ ___ ___   Tuition reimbursement   ___ ___ ___ ___

___ ___ ___ ___   Continuing education opportunities ___ ___ ___ ___

___ ___ ___ ___   Employee assistance programs   ___ ___ ___ ___

___ ___ ___ ___   Day care   ___ ___ ___ ___

___ ___ ___ ___   Leaves of absence   ___ ___ ___ ___

___ ___ ___ ___   Flexible work schedules   ___ ___ ___ ___

How are you two evaluations different? When you look for a job, which list should you use, and why?

End of exercise. Text continues on following page.

fessionals outside of the company that help
:kers with substance abuse problems, stress re-
:tion, and family counseling. The belief is that
sonal or family problems impact the quality of
:k. Correcting these problems helps the em-
yee and the employer.

he number and amount of benefits vary con-
:rably from employer to employer. Sometimes
y vary from employee to employee. This con-
t, often called the cafeteria or shopping cart
thod, allows employees to select from the vari-
benefits offered by the firm. Unmarried em-
yees may wish to exchange dependent insur-
:e for increased personal insurance and so on.
s allows employees to select the benefits that
t suit their needs and situations.

OFIT SHARING

other form of compensation sometimes seen in
lth-care firms is profit sharing. Here the em-
yees share in the productivity and profit of the
1. Profit sharing is intended to provide an
led incentive to workers because they receive
ne of the benefits of the firm's doing well.
netimes profit sharing is paid at the end of the
r. In other instances the money is invested ac-
ding to the employee's wishes and given to him
her upon leaving the company.

mmary

s chapter has introduced general economic
cepts and has applied them to health care and
ployees. Economic principles were covered so
t the environment in which health-care facili-
operate and the way it affects health-care facil-
s could be better understood. This understand-
provides a basis for comprehending the
abilities and limitations health-care facility
ners and managers face. Knowledge of these ca-
bilities and limitations also allows for better un-
standing of what these employers can and can-
t do for employees.

Examining the way economics impacts employ-
provides a basis for comparing the offerings of
ious employers, but, more important, it helps
slain how salaries are set and why. This knowl-
ge can alleviate much of the confusion and mis-

understanding that workers lacking this information often have.

REFERENCES

1. Mansfield, E: Principles of Microeconomics, ed 3. WW Norton, New York, 1980, p 9.
2. Ibid, p 219.
3. Nickson, JW: Economics and Social Choice. McGraw-Hill, New York, 1971, p 28.
4. Pride, W, et al: Business, ed 6. Houghton Mifflin, Boston, 1999, p 10–13.
5. Nickson, p 29.
6. Ibid, p 31.
7. Mansfield, p 441–48.
8. Keynes, JM: The General Theory of Employment, Interest, and Money. Harcourt Brace Jovanovich, New York, 1936.
9. Baumol, W, and Blinder, A: Economics: Principles and Policy. Harcourt Brace Jovanovich, New York, 1979, p 798.
10. Hospitals need leadership. Management Review, December 1990.
11. Nickson,, JW, p 33.
12. Baldor, RA.: Managed Care Made Simple. Blackwell Science, Malden, Mass., 1998, p 7.
13. Ibid, p 3.
14. Ibid, p 2.
15. Ibid, p 8.
16. Lutz, S, et al: Med Inc. Jossey-Bass, San Francisco, 1998.
17. Baldor, RA, pp 10–11.
18. Ibid, pp 41–44.
19. Birenbaum, A: Managed Care: Made In America. Praeger, Westport, Conn., 1997, p 37.
20. Knight, W: Managed care: What It Is and How It Works. Aspen, Gaithersburg, Md., 1998, p 23.
21. Ibid, p 89.
22. Baldor, pp 10–11.
23. Danzi, JT: Positioning Your Practice for the Managed care Market. Williams & Wilkins, Baltimore, Md., 1996, pp 159–60.
24. Baldor, p 14–15.
25. Knight, p 24.
26. Ibid, p 41
27. Ibid, p 46.
28. Mansfield, p 309.
29. Stewart, C, and Siddayao, C: Increasing the Supply of Medical Personnel. Washington, DC, American Enterprise Institute for Public Policy Research, 1973, p 31.
30. Ibid, p 7.
31. Pride, et al, p 260.
32. Berg, JG: Managing Compensation. AMACOM, New York, 1976, pp 116–22.
33. Ibid, pp 123–30.
34. Aldag, R, and Stearns, T: Management. Southwestern Publishing, Cincinnati, 1991, p 321.
35. Aldag and Stearns, p 322.
36. Daft, Richard: Management, ed 5. Dryden, Fort Worth, 2000, pp 417–19.
37. Magid, R: The Work and Family Challenge. New York, American Management Association Membership Publications, 1990, pp 18–19.
38. Pride, et al, pp 258–62.

APPENDIX 4–1

ANSWERS TO BUILDING COMPREHENSION EXERCISE 4–1

Operating a Managed-care Organization (MCO)

In this exercise you will see what it is like to operate a managed care organization. In your MCO, you have 67,000 members, and you allocated $11,000 for each member to cover costs for 1 year. Your task is to calculate costs for each quarter, report on the status of your funds, and make an important decision after the 3rd quarter. (Note: If your calculator does not handle hundreds of millions [9 digits], you may leave off the last 3 digits and calculate everything in thousands of dollars. So 737,000,000 becomes 737,000 thousands [737 million is then 737 thousand thousands]). Items in boldface type are used elsewhere in the exercise.

First, how much money do you have to work with?

$$67,000 \times \$11,000 = \$737,000,000$$

Subtract administrative costs to run the MCO

$$\$737,000,000 - \$66,000,000$$

What is left to pay all of the member medical claims for the year?

$$\textbf{Yearly budget} = \$671,000,000$$

How much can you spend on all of the member medical claims for each quarter?

$$\$671,000,000/ 4 = \$167,750,000$$

Yearly budget divided by 4 = **Quarterly budget**

How much can you spend on each member each quarter?

$$\$167,750,000/ 67,000 = \$2,503.73$$

Quarterly budget divided by 67,000

Now we need to calculate the MCO's financial condition quarter by quarter.

1st Quarter

Enter your Quarterly Budget amount on this line.	$167,750,000
Claims for the 1st Quarter. (Subtract from Quarterly Budget.)	− $107, 669,000
This is the 1st Quarter Budget Variance. Is it positive or negative?	+$60,081,000
What are your Cash Reserves? Enter Yearly Budget figure here.	$671,000,000
Subtract 1st Quarter Claims.	− $107, 669,000
Cash Reserves after the 1st Quarter =	+$563,331,000

2nd Quarter

Enter your Quarterly Budget amount on this line.	$167,750,000
Claims for the 2nd Quarter. (Subtract from Quarterly Budget.)	−$226,393,000
This is the 2nd Quarter Budget Variance. Is it positive or negative?	−$58,643,000
What are your Cash Reserves?	
Enter Cash Reserves after the 1st Quarter here.	+$563,331,000
Subtract 2nd Quarter Claims.	−$226,393,000
Cash Reserves after the 2nd Quarter =	+ $336,938,000

3rd Quarter

Enter your Quarterly Budget amount on this line.	$167,750,000
Claims for the 3rd Quarter. (Subtract from Quarterly Budget.)	−$212,189,000
This is the 3rd Quarter Budget Variance. Is it positive or negative?	−$44,439.000
What are your Cash Reserves?	
Enter Cash Reserves after the 2nd Quarter here.	+ 336,938,000
Subtract 2nd Quarter Claims.	−$212,189,000
Cash Reserves after the 3rd Quarter =	+ $124,749,000

Let's see how things are going.

Compare your Cash Reserves after the 3rd Quarter	+ $124,749,000
to the Quarterly Budget.	−$167,750,000
Subtract the Quarterly Budget from 3rd Quarter Reserves.	−$ 43,001,000

If the result is a positive number, the MCO is doing well. If the result is a negative number, the MCO is not doing well.

4th Quarter

Calculate how much money is left to spend per MCO member.

Enter the Cash Reserves after the 3rd Quarter here.	+ $124,749,000
Divide this by the number of members.	/67,000
The result is how much is left for each member.	$1,861.93

This is also the influenza season. There is a new drug on the market, Outfluenza, which is very effective in minimizing the duration and severity of the flu. However, it must be taken within 8 hours of the first symptoms and then again 8 and 16 hours after the first dose. This means that members need Outfluenza in their homes just in case they think they are starting to get sick. This costs $49 per member for a total of $3,283,000. Do you supply Outfluenza to all MCO members or not?

IF YOU SAID "**YES**" AND BOUGHT ALL MEMBERS OUTFLUENZA USE THESE NUMBERS:

4th Quarter

Enter your Quarterly Budget amount on this line.	$167,750,000
Subtract the cost of Outfluenza.	− $3,283,000
Remaining 4th Quarter Budget.	$164,467,000
Claims for the 4th Quarter. (Subtract from remaining Quarterly Budget.)	−$139,963,000
This is the 4th Quarter Budget Variance. Is it positive or negative?	+ $ 24,504,000
What are your Cash Reserves?	
Enter Cash Reserves after the 3rd Quarter here.	+ $124,749,000
Subtract the cost of Outfluenza.	−$3,283,000
Remaining Cash Reserves.	$121,466,000
Subtract 4th Quarter Claims.	−$139,963,000
Cash Reserves FOR THE YEAR =	−$ 18,497,000

If the Cash Reserves For The Year are positive, you made a profit. If the Cash Reserves For The Year are negative, you lost money.

IF YOU SAID "**NO**" AND DID NOT BUY ALL MEMBERS OUTFLUENZA, USE THESE NUMBERS:

4th Quarter

Enter your Quarterly Budget amount on this line.	$167,750,000
Claims for the 4th Quarter. (Subtract from Quarterly Budget.)	−$249,441,000
This is the 4th Quarter Budget Variance. Is it positive or negative?	−$ 81,691,000
What are your Cash Reserves?	
Enter Cash Reserves after the 3rd Quarter here.	+ $124,749,000
Subtract 4th Quarter Claims.	− $249,441,000
Cash Reserves FOR THE YEAR =	−$124,692,000

If the Cash Reserves For The Year are positive, you made a profit. If the Cash Reserves For The Year are negative, you lost money.

5 • Management: Why It Is Needed; Learning to Live with It

OBJECTIVES

On completion of this chapter, the reader will be able to:

☐ Explain management's role and the manager's job.

☐ Outline the managerial and social forces in the working environment.

☐ List and explain the functions of management.

☐ Identify, describe, and differentiate the two main management styles.

☐ Identify, describe, and differentiate the two organizations that exist in the working environment.

☐ Describe how health workers who have become managers have actually changed careers.

☐ Describe the difficulties facing middle managers.

☐ Explain how managee actions can affect the way a manager treats a managee.

Ask someone what his or her manager does, and a typical reply would be, "Nothing." This seems to be especially true in professional organizations like the health fields where the supervisor or department head is usually a health professional who "advanced" to become a manager. These managers are often seen as fellow professionals who could be "out on the floor working" but who instead are sitting in an office doing "nothing." One of the reasons for the misconception about what managers do comes from a lack of understanding about what management's role really is. Managers rarely, if ever, explain their job to those they manage. Without an explanation it is hard to appreciate someone else's job. Consequently, most people find out what management is like only after they become a manager. This chapter will correct this situation by explaining the role of management, managers, and the people they manage.

To explain the management roles found in most working environments, this chapter will examine management functions, the role of managers, the types of management styles, the formal and informal roles of managers and workers, and the effect workers can have on managers and on coworkers.

Management's Role

The roles of managers and workers are actually recent developments. Before the industrial age the vast majority of people worked alone as farmers, artisans, and craftsmen.[1] They generally owned their own tools and had a variety of skills. There was little need for management because the basic working environment had few employees. There was a relationship between masters and apprentices, but it was more closely related to that of teacher and student than to that of manager and worker. After the Industrial Revolution there were major work environment changes.[2] Then, for the first time, large numbers of people were brought together to work in someone else's building. A means of organizing and controlling these large numbers became necessary. Because *large* numbers of people were involved, the organizing, controlling, directing, and planning could not be accomplished by the owner or by even a few owners. The owner or owners needed to extend themselves. Because they couldn't be in more than one place at a time, they hired others to perform some of the planning, controlling, organizing, and directing. These people were called *managers* to distinguish them from *workers*.

From the beginning a mistake was made in calling the planners, controllers, organizers, and directors *managers* and referring to the people they managed as *workers, subordinates,* or even *employees.* Especially with time, these terms came to imply that *workers* were inferior to or lower than managers. Some places even referred to the two groups as *superiors* and *subordinates,* rather than managers and workers. Not surprisingly, many people thought that if they were the *workers,* were those other people (the managers) *non*workers? The feeling that "subordinates" work and managers do not was one of the factors that led to employment unrest, especially in the 1930s. The charts the managers used to depict the new organizations that they had devised created another

problem. The managers placed themselves above the workers on these organization charts. This design reinforced the message that managers were superior to workers. It also made it seem as if moving into management was a step up—an advancement, or betterment, from the lower position of worker. Actually, moving from being a frontline worker to manager is a change in careers, just as moving from carpentry to health care.

These attitudes still exist today, which complicates the working environment. So it may be time for a new term, especially because most managers are themselves managed. We will use the terms *manager* and *managee* (similar to *franchiser* and *franchisee* or *mortgagor* and *mortgagee*). The term *managee* will mean any person who is managed by someone else. In this way we eliminate the negative connotations of terms like *subordinate,* and move away from the implication that managers do not work.

MANAGEMENT'S WORK WORLD

The current work environment is also affected by the way managers plan, control, organize, and direct work resources. Before the two main methods of managing can be discussed, the functions and resources that comprise management's work world must be examined.

Management has four basic functions: planning, controlling, organizing, and directing.[3] Managers perform these functions with four basic kinds of resources: human, financial, material, and informational.[4] Combining functions and resources results in 16 activities: management must plan for human, financial, material, and informational resources, control human, financial, material, and informational resources, and so on. A particular manager's workweek is not divided into 16 sections, however. A manager could be involved in organizing informational resources when a piece of equipment fails. This development forces him or her to shift to controlling material resources. Although it is possible to manage these 16 areas simultaneously and to concentrate on first one and then another, these functions need to be separated here to make the study and understanding of them possible.

Planning involves the setting of goals. It includes strategic planning, long-term and short-term; setting objectives; and creating operating plans and standard procedures.[5] Managers try to establish as many routines or standard procedures as possible. Managees should be allowed to handle as many of the routine procedures as possible; managers should only be called in when something out of the ordinary happens. During the planning process, some managers may ask for the managee's opinions, but the decision making and prioritizing of company goals is management's domain.

Controlling means overseeing or supervising, disciplining, evaluating, and managing change.[6] The controlling function involves evaluating the performance of managees, measuring the performance of equipment, analyzing the usefulness of information, and controlling the financial resources of the department or institution. Managees may be asked to participate in the evaluation of equipment. Of course, managees should always be involved in their own performance evaluations.

Organizing involves coordinating departmental operations, combining the four resources, forming managee work groups, and creating and staffing the formal organization (the chain of command).[7] Management is responsible for allocating and grouping the four resources to accomplish the goals and objectives of the organization. This includes scheduling working hours, breaks, and lunchtime to meet the needs of the patients or clients and the managees.

Directing involves providing leadership and motivating the workers.[8] Leaders provide vision and direction for the organization. A good leader uses his or her power to inspire people. Providing leadership is not easy, and many good managers are not great leaders.[9]

Motivating people is also not easy and not well understood. If motivation were well understood, there would not be the numerous theories of motivation described in Chapter 9. Motivating managees ranges from providing rewards to simply providing a working environment conducive to self-motivation.[10]

MANAGEMENT ENVIRONMENTS

In carrying out the four functions, managers must contend with two environments: external and internal.

The *external* environment is composed of the political, social, and economic atmosphere, and it is greatly affected by the type of government, both local and national, that is currently in power. An example of the effect the external environment can have on management would be recent attempts at restructuring health care in the United States and instituting national health insurance. The press and the public are also part of the external environment.

The *internal* environment that a manager must contend with is influenced or controlled by the type of ownership the institution has. A public hospital is often managed quite differently from a private, for-profit hospital. The internal environment is also influenced by the type of service being provided, attitudes of the entire work group, attitudes of a manager's direct subordinates, and management style that is being used.

Management Principles

Principles have been developed throughout the history and practice of management to improve the operation of organizations. Understanding these principles can improve your understanding of how organizations function and why organizations are the way they are. The pertinent principles of management that will be discussed here are:

- Division of labor
- Authority
- Unity of command
- Unity of direction
- Hierarchical structure
- Technical competence
- Separation

These are only general principles of management, and some managers do not apply all of them.

The *division of labor principle* is actually very old. It states that great efficiency is obtained when large jobs are divided into component tasks.[11] Each task is then typically performed by one person. For example, the job of removing someone's appendix begins when admitting personnel process the patient and the paperwork. A transporter assists the patient to a hospital room. Nurses provide care before and after surgery. Medical technologists perform laboratory exams. Pharmacists, dietitians, surgeons, anesthesiologists, housekeepers, and others all perform their tasks. Of course, it would be possible for one person to perform all of these tasks, but it would not be very efficient. One person attempting to perform all of these tasks would have to have had extraordinary training, and even then the job would take much longer. It would also be difficult for one person to perform all of these tasks adequately. This is true for a simple operation like an appendectomy. Larger jobs, like open heart surgery, are virtually impossible for one person to perform. The division of labor principle applies to these and other concerns about efficiency (Table 5–1). It is actually the division of labor principle that has created the various health professions and the specialties within each profession.

There are three principles to guide managers in the directing of the four resources. The first is the

TABLE 5–1 • **REASONS FOR THE DIVISION OF LABOR PRINCIPLE**

1. Expertise	Because a person specializes in one area, he or she can become expert in the knowledge and performance of the specialized area.
2. Efficiency	Someone performing the same tasks over and over eventually becomes faster and able to identify and adapt to common problems faster.
3. Time compression	By having a number of specialists performing tasks simultaneously, the total job can be completed faster than if one person had to complete the tasks sequentially.
4. Makes large jobs possible	Some jobs are so large and complex that one person could not complete all of the tasks involved in a reasonable time or in a lifetime.
5. Training	Because specialists require less knowledge than a hypothetical person who knows everything about the medical field and his or her practice, training is faster than it otherwise would be.

authority principle. It states that managers have the right to direct managees to accomplish the goals of the organization and the tasks at hand.[12] Managers may issue orders or simply ask managees to complete tasks. In either case, it is the manager who ultimately decides who will do what, when, where, and how. On the other hand, managers are then responsible for getting the tasks accomplished. With the manager's right to tell managees what to do comes the responsibility for achieving, or failing to achieve, the goals of the organization. Much of a manager's job is being responsible for those he or she manages.

The second guide for managers in directing people is the *unity of command principle.* This principle states that managees should report to only one boss.[13] In this use of the term, *unity* is derived from unit, meaning *one,* rather than from united, implying a collectivity. Although each manager may have many managees, each managee should be receiving direction from only one immediate supervisor. Otherwise, there is a very great potential for someone to receive conflicting orders from two bosses. Although in many industries the unity of command principle is practiced, the health-care industry is often not one of them. Typically, health-care managees answer to an administrative manager (one from the same health profession) and to a physician. This violation of the unity of command principle is usually handled by having the physician be responsible for medical decisions, while having the administrative manager be responsible for organizational or managerial decisions.

The third guiding fundamental for the directing function is the *unity of direction principle.* This principle states that tasks that are similar and tasks that work toward achieving the same organizational goal should be grouped under one manager.[14] Hospitals are an excellent example of this principle being put into practice. If hospitals were organized by function only, there would be a manager for radiographers, a manager for receptionists, a manager for medical transcriptionists (some of whom transcribe radiology reports), a manager for transporters, and so on. Following the unity of direction principle allows for one manager to supervise radiographers and radiology department receptionists, transcribers, and transporters. Rather than grouping people strictly by what they do (by function), the unity of direction principle provides a basis for grouping all the people that are working toward the goal of providing diagnostic radiology services together.

These three principles—authority, unity of command, and unity of direction—account for much of the structure of organizations. They account for so much of the structure that together they help to form another principle, the *hierarchical structure principle.* This principle states that a hierarchy, or chain of command, is needed to provide direction and control for individuals and the organization (Fig. 5–1).[15] Both control and direction begin at the top of the pyramidlike structure and travel throughout the organization. This structure allows for large organizations to act as one and helps to ensure that the areas, or departments, within an organization work with, and not against, each other.

The last two principles that will be examined here concern the staffing of organizations and the relationship between an organization and the people that comprise it. The first is the *technical competence principle,* and although it sounds as though it has come from contemporary concerns for discrimination, it actually dates from the late 19th and early 20th centuries. The technical competence principle states that people should be hired and assigned work according to their abilities.[16] Hiring and assignments should be made on rational terms—the best performer should receive the assignment. No consideration should be given to the liking, preferences, family relationships, or prejudices of the manager. By following this principle,

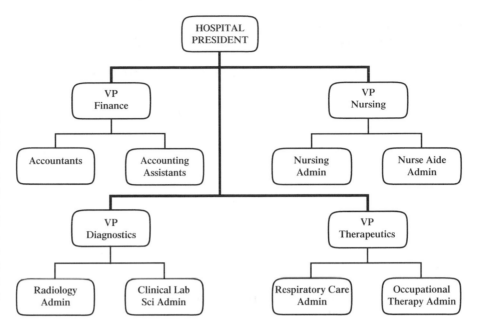

FIGURE 5–1 • The Hierarchical Structure Principle. The principle states that a hierarchy, or chain of command, is needed to provide direction and control for individuals and the organization. The boxes represent positions in the organization. The lines are the formal lines of communication. The chart also reveals the departments or the organization. Both control and direction begin at the top of the pyramidlike structure and travel throughout the organization.

managers are supposed to be able to maximize the performance of the organization.

The *separation principle* has its origins in ancient times when nepotism was prevalent. It is also a simply stated principle that has a wide-ranging effect. The separation principle states that a position in an organization is separate from the person in the position.[17] If John Doe is a manager, he is separate from the managerial position he is filling. The separation principle creates two distinct entities: the position in an organization and the person filling the position.

To comply with the separation and technical competence principles, managers created job descriptions and job specifications. *Job descriptions* represent the positions in the organization and include information such as the tasks associated with the position, the responsibilities, the working conditions, and the equipment that will be used. *Job specifications* depict the personal characteristics needed to fulfill the job description. The job specification would describe the education, work experience, acquired skills, and physical abilities needed to perform in the position outlined in the job description. Theoretically, managers take a job specification and find people that fit it. The person that best meets the specification is then, theoretically, the best person to hire for the position. How well the person performs is then measured with a performance appraisal that is derived from the job specification (Fig. 5–2).

Knowing the basic principles that form the foundation of management methods can help you understand how and why organizations and managers function the way they do. In addition to these basic principles, there are two general methods managers

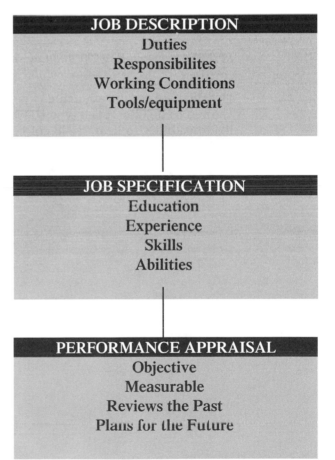

FIGURE 5–2 • Job descriptions explain the position—the job itself. Job specifications describe the qualifications a person would need to be able to perform the tasks listed in the job description. The performance appraisal then measures how well the person with the qualifications listed in the job specification is performing the tasks listed in the job description. Job descriptions are created before job specifications; performance appraisal forms are then created after job specifications.

 Building Comprehension Exercise begins on following page

BUILDING COMPREHENSION EXERCISE 5–1

Developing Job Descriptions and Specifications

Part A: Create a job description for a person in your profession.

1. List the duties an entry-level worker would perform.

2. Identify any duties that are responsibilities and move them to this section. Responsibilities are different from duties in that if someone fails to perform a duty, it can be repeated without causing great harm or loss. If one fails to perform a responsibility, simply repeating the activity does not really correct the situation. In health care, examples of responsibilities would include handling medicine or maintaining sterile fields.

3. List typical working conditions. This refers to the days and times one works, holidays, travel, etc.

4. List the types of tools or equipment one must be able to use.

Part B: Create a job specification for the position you just described.

List the type of education and experience needed. Skills refer to things one must have learned to do, like touch type 60 words per minute. Abilities refer to physical capabilities, like the ability to hear, see in color, lift 40 lb from the floor to a 4-ft high shelf 30 times an hour.

End of exercise. Text continues on following page.

use when applying the principles and when performing the four management functions on the four managerial resources: classical and behavioral.

Classical Management

Two basic schools of management theory exist: classical and behavioral. They are not dichotomous, however. Rather, they form two extremes with many variations between. Of the two, classical management is the older theory.

Classical management was the first system to evolve.[18] Knowing how it came about is important to understand current management thought and the behavior of many untrained managers. Classical management developed along with the Industrial Revolution, accelerating near the end of the 19th century. Before this time most people worked essentially alone. The working environment of the Industrial Revolution was the first time large groups of people came together under one roof to use other people's (the owner's) equipment to perform work. Because this practice was so new, there were no managerial methods to apply. Early managers had only three examples on which to base their theories. Before the Industrial Revolution the only institutions that organized large numbers of people were the armed forces, churches, and slavery. All three used similar autocratic methods. Thus early management systems were similarly autocratic.

The system that began to form, which was later called *classical management* and which is still in use today, was a *command system*. Its basic components are a chain of command (see Fig. 5–1) and a system where "superiors" give orders (or commands) to "subordinates."[19] Superiors and subordinates are in quotation marks because, as mentioned earlier, there is nothing inherently better about the superiors, nor is their work of greater value (in fact, if it were not for the subordinates, the superiors would have no one to manage and nothing to do). Superiors are simply higher up on the chain of command.

Actually, early management systems evolved into autocratic, command systems for three main reasons:

1. Early management thought was influenced by other examples of command systems that had existed previously.[20] At the time, the only examples for organizing large numbers of people were military organizations and religious organizations.[21] Both used a hierarchical system of controls that flowed down from a single leader, just as they do today. It is easy to see how an early industrial-era business owner could see himself in the position of a general, admiral, or the pope. Middle managers assumed the positions from colonel, captain, lieutenant, ensign, and bishop monsignor, priest. Following these examples included keeping decision making and power at the top of the organization. Orders were issued, sent down the chain of command, and were expected to be obeyed.

2. The command system seemed to be the most logical approach.[22] The managers and owners believed that the most straightforward, expedient way to get workers to do something was to tell them to do it. If you had three different tasks, it seemed to make sense that you tell one group to do this, and another to do that, and the third group gets to do everything else. Simple. And because the people giving the orders were either owners or managers working on behalf of the owners, they did not see any reason why the workers should be included in the order giving and decision making. It also did not seem important whether the workers liked being told what to do or not. This was a simple exchange. The owner gave you money, and you gave him work. And if you didn't like it, you could always quit.

3. The workforce was much less educated and essentially inexperienced.[23] Because the education level of the workforce was so low and because many of the jobs created during the Industrial Revolution did not exist before, workers *had* to be told what to do. They possessed neither the knowledge nor the experience to manage themselves.

As the Industrial Revolution progressed, the knowledge and experience of owners, managers, and workers advanced. Eventually the command methods were modified and codified. One of the first to develop management thought into an integrated system was Fredrick Taylor.

Taylor[24] devised a way to apply the scientific method to the workplace, and he called his classical system of management *scientific management*. Taylor was convinced that he could find through experimentation the one best way to perform every job. In doing so, he sought to improve productivity and conditions and wages for workers. For example, Taylor would study the moving or loading of heavy barrels or boxes and devise improved methods for doing the work. This was good for management, and more often than not the new way would be less tiresome for the managee or place less strain on his back or prove to be safer. Scientific management was also responsible for coffee breaks. It was found that a managee could accomplish more by being given periodic breaks than by working 8 hours nonstop. There were also negative aspects for the workers, however. One was that after the "one best way" had been established, all managees were expected follow it.[25] There was little room given for personal variations or innovations.

Today the classical system has these characteristics:

- An emphasis on the manager.
- The manager is responsible for the success of the organization, rather than the managees. The manager's skill at selecting and motivating the right managees enables the organization to function efficiently.
- An autocratic style.
- Explicit managee directions.
- Control of as much of the work environment as possible.
- Little management consideration for managee attitudes or morale.
- Little managee freedom.
- An assumption that most managees are lazy, and, if left on their own, would choose not to work.
- Money as the main, or the only, motivator.
- An emphasis on downward communication.
- An emphasis on the chain of command.[26–29]

There are two other factors to consider when contemplating whether to apply classical management theories.

The first consideration involves situations in which the application of classical management is particularly effective.[30] For positions requiring low levels of skill, education, and experience, classical management is the method of choice. These situations are similar to the conditions prevalent during the Industrial Revolution. In addition, the alternative management style (behavioral management—discussed in the following section) cannot be used because it requires a high level of involvement by the managees. In low-skill positions, managees are usually unable to participate even if they are willing. Thus, with low-skill positions, the command system appears to work best.

The second consideration for the application of classical management involves the managees. Some managees simply do not wish to participate in their own management or in the decision-making process. Both are required if behavioral management is to be used. Sometimes whole groups of managees do not wish to participate or are re-

stricted from doing so by labor or union contract arrangements. Other times it may be that one person in the group has an attitude or a personality trait that requires close supervision. Some people perform their share of the work on their own; some will do as little as they are allowed. The latter types often force a manager to treat them differently.[31] They receive more scrutiny, but they bring it on themselves.

Finally, it is important to keep in mind that classical management represents one extreme point of view. The other extreme, behavioral management, will be discussed next, as will the relationship between the two. For now, suffice it to say that some managers are devotedly classical and some situations require classical management. Other managers are only somewhat classical, whereas other situations require the use of some classical management principles and some behavioral management principles.[32]

Behavioral Management

As organizations became more complex and front-line workers became better trained and educated, the need for an alternative to classical management began to develop.[33] Workers' initial dissatisfaction with the way management treated them resulted in small rebellions. The workers, however, had few rights, and these rebellions were often put down by physical force or the firing of workers or both.[34] Two responses to classical management and to the developmental and educational advances of workers emerged. Workers responded by forming unions, and worker rights were established by law.[35,36] Managers developed behavioral management, but in a circuitous way, for *behavioral,* or *participative, management* began as a typical scientific management study.

In the 1920s, Western Electric performed a series of experiments at its Hawthorne plant in Cicero, Illinois. The experiments were designed to study the effects of changes in the physical work environment on productivity.[37] Prior to the experiments, managees at the Hawthorne plant assembled telephone equipment at anonymous workstations in a large assembly room. For purposes of the experiments and to satisfy the needs of a scientific study, two work groups were formed. Each group worked in a separate room. One group was the control group. Conditions in the room of the control group would not be changed. The other group was the experimental group. In the experimental room environmental factors would be changed to determine what effect, if any, each change had on productivity. For example, the intensity of the room lighting was changed. As the lights got brighter, productivity in the experimental room increased. However, productivity in the control room also increased, yet there the lighting had not changed. Then the lighting was decreased in the experimental room. It continued to decrease until the researchers found the level at which the assemblers could no longer work. Here were other unexpected results. Up to the point where the workers could no longer see to assemble their parts, productivity *increased*. The researchers had assumed that as the lights got brighter, productivity might increase, and as they got dimmer, productivity would decrease. Instead, it increased. Productivity also increased in the control group, and there the lighting did *not* decrease. Clearly, something unusual was happening.

The researchers re-examined what had happened. Ideally, a scientific experiment alters only one factor. If a change is produced (and others can duplicate what has been done), a cause-and-effect relationship can be established. It is concluded that the alteration produced the change. The Hawthorne experiments were confusing not because of the changes in the experimental group—it was expected that there would be an effect on productivity. The challenge was to explain the unexpected increases in productivity in the control group. For answers the researchers called on an Australian professor from Harvard University. Elton Mayo brought in a team that studied the Hawthorne experiments for 4 years before they determined that something other than the environmental changes caused the increases in productivity in the two groups. Maybe the Hawthorne studies demonstrated that environmental factors do not affect productivity. Or maybe something in addition to the environmental factors had been inadvertently changed. After much consideration, Mayo and his team concluded that the conducting of the experiment and the researchers themselves had an effect on the results.

Up until this time no one had taken much notice of what these individual Hawthorne assembly workers did. They had been supervised, but this was the first time someone was interested in their work *and* this was the first time anyone told them how they were doing on a regular basis. What changed the productivity in both rooms were the creation of work groups with whom the members could identify, the attention given to the managees and their work by the researchers, the managees' feelings that they were doing something important, and the constant feedback the managees received on their performance. Thus was behavioral management born. Now managers believed

that treating managees well and letting them know when they are doing well improves productivity. The researchers at Hawthorne had discovered that there is more to work than performing a task for money.

Behavioralism also arose from the mismanagement of the human element of work by the classical system.[38] Behavioral managers believe that a satisfied, involved managee is a better worker.[39] Behavioral managers also feel that the survival of the company is a responsibility of everyone in the organization. They realize that not only can frontline workers have ideas about their jobs, but often they are in the best position to make suggestions for change. Other characteristics of behavioral management include:

- Advocating the social, as well as the economic, output of work
- Recognizing the managee's ability to think and contribute ideas to the workplace
- Allowing as much managee self-determination as possible
- Trying to make every job a learning experience for the managee and practicing job enrichment and job enlargement techniques
- Emphasizing upward as well as downward communication
- Recognizing the informal organization
- Managers' being viewed as leaders of a work group rather than overseers
- Managees' being seen as wanting to work and being capable of enjoying work

Behavioralists, and situations in which behavioral management is applicable, require more participation from managees in decision making and working conditions than classical management does. Behavioralists are more likely to listen to managee feedback and act on it.[40] Behavioral managers place a greater emphasis on communicating with the workers in their departments. They also understand that the managees have an existence beyond the workplace and that sometimes peoples' private lives affect their work both positively and negatively.[41] Behavioralists also believe that every job should be a learning experience and that managees' abilities should grow as part of the job.[42] Last, a *major* difference between classical and behavioral managers is that true behavioralists are willing to share power and decision-making authority with their managees.[43] Behavioral managers believe that they and their managees are part of a team; the managers just happen to do a somewhat different job than the managees.

The Management Continuum

Few managers are 100 percent classical or 100 percent behavioral. These two systems are not so much separate entities as they are the extreme ends of a continuum (Fig. 5–3). Most managers fall somewhere between the two ends. Some are very classical, and some are very behavioral. Some lean toward the classical end, whereas others are nearer the behavioral side. Actually, a *professional manager* is one who has been educated as a situational manager—one who can use any combination of the two methods depending on the type of management a particular situation calls for. As an example, ditch digging does not lend itself to total behavioralism. Basically a supervisor tells one person to dig there and another to dig here. He tells them how deep, wide, and long to dig and to not hit each other with a shovel. There is not much need for a discussion or for participative management. On the other, a manager cannot walk into a room filled with physicists and say, "Discover the laws that explain the combined electromagnetic weak force, the strong nuclear force, and the gravitational force by Friday at 3:00 pm." Jobs that call for creativity must be performed in a management climate with more latitude in determining work rules. People who perform work that must be uniform with the work of others or who cannot be trusted to contribute a full day's work require closer supervision. Because situations vary and because strengths and weaknesses vary among individuals, management styles must be chosen with flexibility and sensitivity.

Management for Health Care

A management style close to the middle of the management continuum is most appropriate for health care. There are two major reasons for this. One is the need for uniformity, and the other is the need to adapt. Health-care managers and workers need to use a blend of classical and behavioral techniques for the good of the patients, workers, and health-care system in general.

The need for uniformity in care and treatment plans, diagnostic procedures and products, and therapies is vital for health care. These plans, products, and therapies must be based on sound scientific principles. Health care must also be as consistent as humanly achievable to ensure the best possible outcome for all patients. In this regard, the management style must be more classically oriented. There must be a procedure manual, and everyone must follow it. Otherwise, there will be no way to predict results, and the benefits of successful approaches will not be available to all.

On the other hand, each patient and each ailment is somewhat different. Health-care workers are educated to be able to identify small and large variations from normal. They must then be free to employ adaptations with certain limits. Health-care workers must also be able to recognize situations that are beyond the limits of the adaptations they may employ. They must then know when to seek assistance rather than force a situation into conformity. Here, a more behavioral approach is needed.

Behavioral management is also needed to help reduce the costs of health care. In this respect, all employees must feel that they are part of the cost-saving team. If workers do not feel they are part of the same team as management, they will feel less responsible to hold down costs and reduce waste.

The Formal Organization

To coordinate the efforts of the people in any work group so that the group's goals and objectives are met, an organizing structure is created. Thus, in typical business enterprises, people within a department are grouped, and then departments are grouped. The result is the *Formal Organization* (see Fig. 5–1) or chain of command. The name and the

Classical Management	Behavioral Management
Authoritarian	Participative
Manager-centered	Managee-centered
Manager makes decisions	Team/group decisions
Focus on the formal organization	Formal and informal organizations recognized

FIGURE 5–3 • The descriptions in the text of classical management and behavioral management refer to two extremes of the same continuum. Few managers are totally classical or totally behavioral. Most managers fall somewhere in between. So they may be very classical or a little classical, very behavioral or a little behavioral, or right between the two extremes.

structure reveal much about management style and terminology.

The chain of command takes its name and much of its function from the command system of human cooperation (see Chap. 4). This helps explain why management styles lean toward the classical system in so many organizations. The very structure lends itself toward the issuing of orders (commands) *from* the managers *to* the managees. Communications pass from "above" to the "lower" levels. This stressing of downward communication further enhances the manager's position because he or she becomes the possessor of information and, therefore, power. The manager *may* or *may not* convey this information to others. The formal organization also depicts the differentiation between managers and managees.

The chain of command structure emphasizes the manager (and de-emphasizes the managee) by placing managers "above" the managees. Furthermore, employees "move up" or "advance" to management, implying that to become a manager is to improve oneself. New managees are often asked about their future plans and are expected to demonstrate motivation and ambition by saying that in 5 years they want to be in a supervisory capacity. But is being a manager or supervisor actually "a step up"? Is it inherently better to be a manager than a worker? The answer is no. In fact, frontline workers are far more vital to any organization than are managers. Without managers but with frontline workers, the business would survive far longer than it would with managers but without frontline workers. Without workers, managers have no purpose.

What then is management if it is not a "step up" from the front lines? What have supervisors done if they have not "advanced"? People who have moved from positions as frontline workers to positions in management have actually changed careers. They are no longer physical therapists, medical technologists, or medical transcriptionists. They are now supervisors or managers. They have changed professions. This sometimes causes problems when managees continue to view a former colleague not as a manager but as a respiratory therapist who could be helping with the workload. The managees see someone who, by definition, is not a worker, so what they are doing is not work.

Classical management relies on the defined structure of the formal organization. This is not meant to imply that behavioral managers do not have a formal organization. They do have a formal, defined structure, but they use it differently than do classical managers. In addition, behavioral management recognizes and employs the informal organization.

The Informal Organization

The formal organization is an orderly, well-defined system that outlines the reporting structure of a company. Almost all are a form of the command system. The organization chart profiles staff relationships within the formal organization and is a diagram of the way things are ideally supposed to be. The reality, of course, is never quite as clear-cut. In contrast, the informal organization reflects the relationships in the organization as they really are.[44]

Every company has a formal and an informal organization.[45] The *informal organization* reflects the true way power is distributed. It takes into account the fact that some bosses like some people more than others, that some people's personalities are stronger than others, that some people are more cooperative than others, and that some people are more outspoken than others. Perhaps most important, the informal organization takes into account the fact that some people are more knowledgeable than others. In short, the informal organization reveals the social nature of the working environment.[46]

The informal organization exists with, and in spite of, the formal organization. The formal organization is like a trellis—orderly and rigid. The informal organization is like a vine that grows randomly on the trellis. It needs the substance and form of the trellis as a base, even though it will not conform exactly to its shape. The informal organization can also be charted like the formal organization, although it rarely is.

Figure 5–4 represents the formal organization in an actual hospital radiology department. After careful observation of the functioning of the department and interviews with the staff, it was possible to create a chart of the informal organization (Fig. 5–5). This chart, sometimes referred to as a *contact chart,* reveals many of the facets of the informal organization.[47] First of all, the position of chief radiographer was vacant. One of the most interesting aspects of the informal organization is its ability to adapt to various situations.[48] In this case, a void was created that had to be filled. The informal organization filled the void automatically by establishing the formally unrecognized position that I had called the "senior radiographer." The informal organization took up the slack left by a vacancy in the formal organization. This can also happen when a manager is weak, inefficient, or ineffective. This adaptability of the informal organization is also what allows departments to function with fewer than the normal number of managees (at least for a short time).

 Building Comprehension Exercise begins on following page

Charting the Formal Organization

Draw the formal organization where you currently work or for your clinical site (if you are assigned to one). If it is available to you, use the organization chart feature of Microsoft Word (click Insert, Object, and select MS Organization Chart from the list on the Create New tab) for an easy way to create neat boxes and lines.

End of exercise. Text continues on following page.

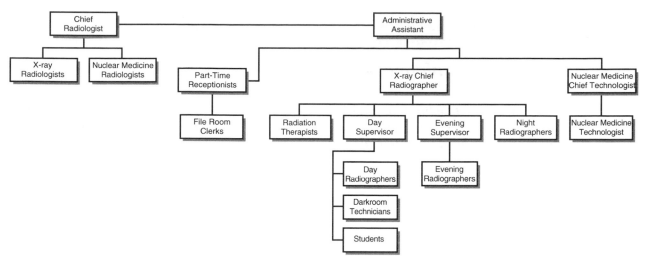

FIGURE 5–4 • The formal organization in an actual hospital radiology department. After careful observation of the functioning of the department and interviews with the staff, it was possible to create a chart of the informal organization.

Other items of interest in these charts are that the evening supervisor and evening radiographers reported to two different people. They reported to the administrative assistant for the 2 hours during which their shifts overlapped, but during the remainder of their shifts, they worked under the emergency department physician.

Another very common situation outlined here is that not all of the radiographers reported to the same persons. Factions, or cliques, seem almost inevitable when more than two people work together, and these are also parts of the informal organization.

In terms of management, it is the behavioralists who recognize and work with the formal and the informal organizations. Strictly classical managers

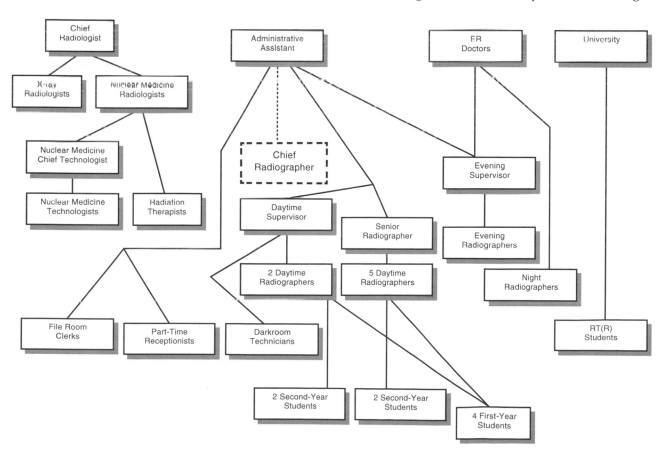

FIGURE 5–5 • This chart reveals many of the facets of the informal organization.

 Building Comprehension Exercise begins on following page

BUILDING COMPREHENSION EXERCISE 5–3

Charting the Informal Organization

After completing Building Comprehension Exercise 5–2, try to determine what the informal organization is like. Who goes to whom for guidance when there is a question? Draw the contact chart and compare it to the formal organization chart. How are they different? Why are they different?

End of exercise. Text continues on following page.

often try to ignore or actively repress the informal organization. The behavioralists recognize that people come to work for more than money; they come for social reasons. Behavioralists believe that the informal organization can be a valuable asset for addressing social and work problems or that it can be a liability if ignored.

As a liability, informal organizations can slow the function of a department either temporarily or by reining in *rate busters* (people working faster than the others, the fear being that management will discover that the job can be done faster and will require everyone to produce at a higher rate).[49] The informal organization can resist change, decrease the effectiveness of the organization, or even push to have a manager replaced (see the following section, "The Middle Manager's Dilemma").[50]

As an asset, the informal organization can contribute ideas to the company, make up for shortcomings in the chain of command, aid the company in times of trouble, and take part in decision making.

As a managee, you will be part of the formal and informal organizations. Your role in the formal organization will probably be well-defined by a job description. Your role in the informal organization will not. Initially you will have no position. During the first days on a new job, the other workers will be evaluating you socially and personally. They will be looking to see if you will be a good worker. This takes into account your job knowledge, dependability, and personality. In general, people like and respect those who are very knowledgeable about their profession, do their share of work (and a little bit more), are extroverted, are from the same socioeconomic background as themselves, and have the same values as the existing group.[51] Breaking into the informal organization is one of the things that most people do not like about starting a new job.

The Middle Manager's Dilemma

Just for a moment imagine yourself in this situation:

You are the supervisor of four employees. Your boss says you must get these people to do three things:

1. Work overtime.
2. Work faster.
3. Improve the quality of their work.

You have called a meeting of these four people to explain the situation. Write down what you would say to these people to accomplish the task your boss has given you.

Next, assume that you made your presentation to these managees, and they all responded with reasons why they could *not* meet these requirements. They couldn't work overtime because they had children to care for, another job, or social lives to attend to. They all thought that they were working as fast as they could. In fact, they thought they were being overworked and that more help was needed in this department. As far as the quality of their work was concerned, they thought it was the best it could be, given that they already thought they were overworked. They felt that if they were to work faster, quality would decrease rather than increase. Now what do you say? Oh, by the way, there is currently a shortage of health workers in your area, so you *cannot* fire them.

Considering the type of people you have to deal with, your second set of arguments will probably fail also. Now your boss wants a progress report. What are you going to tell him or her? How will you explain that you cannot get these managees to meet those three goals? What are you going to do when your boss reminds you that it is much easier to replace one supervisor (you!) than it is to replace an entire department full of managees? This is the middle manager's dilemma.

The middle manager's dilemma can be described as being caught between a rock and a hard spot. Middle managers must deal with orders from the managers above them and the preferences of the managees below them. It is not easy. They receive pressure from both sides, often carrying out directives that they have had little input toward developing or that they do not agree with and managing people whom they did not hire. This creates a difficult situation for the manager and the managees.

The Managee's Role

How does the worker, the managee, fit into the organizational and managerial systems just described? The managee is the most important component of the organization. Workers are the sole reason for the existence of organization structures. Because of the complexity of modern organizations and the need for expert knowledge in the performance of individual tasks in the accomplishment of larger goals, there is a need for people other than frontline workers.

Frontline workers, managees, are needed to perform the individual tasks that comprise the overall goals of organizations. In the health-care professions, different people, each expert at a particular job, are needed to maintain people's health or to return them to good health. It would be virtually impossible for one person to admit a patient, monitor and care for the patient, clean the patient's room, prepare and deliver the patient's meals, perform numerous diagnostic tests, prepare medications, deliver medications, apply treatments, manage therapies, issue bills, collect money, monitor equipment and the physical plant, and pay everyone. The depth of knowledge required is too great. So there are specialties and subspecialties. There are specialists for performing the health functions and specialists for the nonhealth functions. There are specialists for planning, controlling, organizing, and directing the human, financial, informational, and material resources of the organization. This complexity creates the manager and managee roles and defines them.

A managee's role, then, is to perform the technical tasks of his or her specialty to the best of his or her abilities and at an acceptable level, while using the least amount of the organization's resources possible. "Performing the technical tasks of his or her specialty" refers to the profession for which you have been educated. These technical tasks need to be performed to best of your ability, but this must also be at an acceptable level. A person cannot be retained if his or her best performance is below adequate. On the other hand, the minimal level of the acceptable performance should not be viewed as the maximum level of performance. If your best performance is better than someone else's, then you must perform at this higher level. There are three reasons for this:

1. People must perform at the highest level possible for them because the opposite action would prove ruinous. If everyone worked at a minimal level or did not work at all, society and our civilization would first stagnate and then collapse. Everyone must try to do his or her best at all times for everyone to progress and prosper. Furthermore, the fact that we have created a society, a situation in which everyone depends on everyone else's work, requires each person to do his or her share.

2. Doing your best is part of our society's work ethic. That ethic states that each person must give "a fair day's work for a fair day's pay."[52] To do less is to cheat the system, which often results in the cheater's being removed from the system (fired).

3. Performing at the highest level possible is the best way to advance. Doing your best is not only right morally and ethically, but the best personal strategy for advancing your career.

People who perform only the minimum may survive, but their chances to flourish and prosper are not great.

In many organizations the frontline worker's role begins and ends with the performance of the technical tasks in his or her profession. The division of labor principle may be followed to the extent that others (managers) are solely responsible for planning, controlling, organizing, directing, and decision making concerning the resources of the organization. Some organizations apply the division of labor principle differently. Behaviorally managed organizations typically involve frontline workers in the managerial and decision-making function of the organization. Some workers want to concentrate on the technical aspects of their profession. They are content with managers' attending to the four functions and the four resources. Other people want to participate in the operations of the organization. Neither is better nor worse, and most organizations function with both types of workers. The knowledge provided in this book will help you to identify organizations and seek out some and avoid others according to your preference.

Self-management

Self-management is an emerging trend as ideas like empowerment and reductions in employees have come to include middle managers. Self-management includes delegating supervisory duties to workers and training in self-management and time management. Training is possibly the most important item for implementing self-management. Workers and managers must have a thorough understanding of what is expected of them, and new workers must be carefully selected and trained in self-management techniques.[53]

COMPONENTS OF SELF-MANAGEMENT

Self-management has five main components. To be self-managing you must (1) be self-directing, (2) be able to apply job redesign to your work, (3) be self-controlling, (4) be self-monitoring and reporting, and (5) be self-rewarding. The application of self-management techniques is designed to make workers as self-sufficient as is feasible. The five components of self-management must also be integrated with one another, but they are also described here in roughly the same order in which they would be performed.

Self-direction consists of setting your own goals and objectives.[54] This sometimes means *redesigning your job* by suggesting changes to your work, the workflow, or the work systems.[55] The power to consider and conduct job redesign fits with self-management and empowerment. How can you manage yourself without the ability to change what you do?

The next step in the process of self-management is *self-control*, which is the regulation of work by the individual.[56] With self-control the individual sets the pace and scheduling of the work that needs to be accomplished to meet the goals and objectives he or she set in earlier stages of self-management. During the self-control phase, tasks are organized—large tasks are divided into smaller and easier to handle elements, deadlines are set, and resources are allocated. One of the most important of these resources is time. Time management is not unique to self-management, but it is a key part of it and will be discussed separately.

Once someone sets goals and establishes a schedule, the next step is *self-monitoring and reporting*. The overall goal of this part of self-management is for the individual to ascertain how well he or she is doing without having to rely on feedback from a manager.[57] Self-monitoring includes self-observation and self-assessment. Reporting involves self-assessment and documentation. In self-observation, the individual monitors and records activities and gathers information on performance toward the completion of goals and objectives.[58] Self-assessment encompasses evaluating the information collected during self-observation.[59]

During self-assessment it is important to determine why some things work and why others sometimes do not. Knowing why things work helps people repeat successful strategies. Understanding why other things do not work helps people change future behavior. Finally, in the documentation step, the results of the self-assessment are reported. Much of this documentation is for the use of the self-managed person. The self-monitoring and reporting component isn't sent to a manager who passes judgment and hands out rewards. That might lead to exaggeration of achievements and hiding of failures. In self-management, self-monitoring and reporting lead to the next step, self-reward.

During the *self-rewarding* step, rewards are received or withheld depending on the completion of specific goals.[60] These rewards might be the ability to take a break or a vacation.[61] The important point is that the individual set and applied the reward. Although self-rewarding can include withholding rewards or administering punishment, there is some opinion that punishments are not as effective as rewards for changing behaviors.[62]

IMPLEMENTING SELF-MANAGEMENT

A number of actions should be taken by organizations so that self-management has a fair chance to succeed. The mission of the organization must be clear, and self-managed workers must clearly understand their jobs.[63,64] Both of these conditions are common in allied health professions. Organizations must also remove barriers to self-management, which is no small task.[65] To do so, training in self-management and allowing time for people to perform self-management tasks are critical.

With these actions, and support from those who will be self-managed, significant increases in productivity and job satisfaction can be realized. However, self-management and other forms of management may owe much of their success or failure to how well or how poorly people manage one key resource—time.

TIME MANAGEMENT

Time is the one resource that we all possess in an equal amount. How we spend the limited time we have can be the factor that separates the more successful from the less successful. The advice "Work smarter, not harder" has been around for some time, and what it really refers to is using time more efficiently. Time management is the way to accomplish much in a short amount of time, and once you learn how to spend your time most wisely, the lesson tends to stay with you for life. Good time management can increase your productivity, and increased productivity can increase your self-esteem.[66]

It needs to be mentioned at the beginning that there is no one best time management method; any method that works for you is good.[67] If you already have a system, the information here may help you refine it. Whether you use a yellow legal pad, sticky notes, a pocket calendar, or a palmtop computer, one thing is certain—any system is better than no system.

Before selecting or creating a time-management system for yourself, you should measure how your time is currently being spent. Completing Building Comprehension Exercise 5–4, "Analyzing Your Time Management Techniques," will help you do this. Then you can examine time-management tips and a discussion on handling big jobs. A cautionary

 Building Comprehension Exercise begins on following page

BUILDING COMPREHENSION EXERCISE 5–4

Analyzing Your Time-management Techniques

One method for determining how you are spending your time is to use a time log. A time log is a sheet (or series of sheets) on which you record how you spend your time each day. (See the following example.) When starting a time log, you should first write down your activities to determine which categories would be most useful to you. Recording the time spent on each category should be done for at least 1 week, although you may have to use the log for 2, 3, 4, or more weeks, depending on your situation. After the time logs have been completed, total the numbers for each activity and calculate the percentage of time spent in each area. This information must then be combined with other information, such as which tasks are not being completed on time. After you know how your time is being spent and what is not getting done, you may employ some of the time-management techniques to gain more control over your time.

Date _____	Work = done on time	Breaks	Driving	Home
Scheduled activities				
Phone				
Looking for misplaced items				
Unplanned visitors				
Redoing previous work/ correcting errors				

End of exercise. Text continues on following page.

note though: Don't create or use a system that takes more time to use than the time it saves you. If, after you learn a system, you find yourself dedicating large amounts of time to writing and rewriting lists and setting priorities, and making different lists, then maybe it is time to consider a simpler system.

Your Peak Time

One of the first steps you can take to work smarter is to find your peak time. Peak time is the hours of the day (or night) when you are most productive. For some people this is early morning. Others don't function well early in the day. (Some feel any time before noon is early.) My peak time has always been between 7:00 PM and midnight. If you are not sure when your peak times are, you may need to develop awareness for the signs of peak and nonpeak times. If difficult tasks consistently seem easier and are completed faster in the morning, then morning is probably your peak time. If you stare at a report or read a sentence over and over and still can't remember what it says, when you tend to slump forward and your forehead bounces off your desk, or if you find your coworkers checking to see if you still have a pulse at 5:30 PM every day, then this is probably not a peak time for you. Whatever your peak times are, find them and try to adjust your schedule so that you perform more demanding tasks during those times.[68] At work, for example, you might schedule routine tasks, meetings, and phone calls for nonpeak times. You then save your peak times for more demanding tasks like analyzing, writing, doing computations, and performing creative work.

Time-management Tips

Once you know your peak times, it is time to start organizing your work. First, you will almost certainly need to find a calendar and time schedule that works for you (and doesn't take more time than it is worth). No matter what you choose, the key is to force yourself to use it until it becomes a habit. You can choose desk calendars, pocket calendars, or appointment books or simply use a legal pad to write a list of things to do that day or week. Or, you can choose one of the many palmtop computers (for example, a Palm m100). Once you have a calendar you are comfortable with, you can schedule your work and allocate times for each task.

Schedule recurring events at the start of a time period. If you have a staff meeting every 2 weeks on Friday for the whole year, then start at the beginning of the year and schedule it in. Or start at the beginning of the quarter or the month, or whatever time period works for you. Assign time for each event, leaving time between events for breaks or events that may go beyond the scheduled time. If you have to prepare for an event, work backward from the due date and give yourself plenty of warning to begin the task. If it will take 2 days to prepare for a meeting, you may need 4 to 6 days' warning in case other things come up.

Once recurring meetings are scheduled, you should block out certain times for other kinds of tasks.[69] You may want to have a callback hour—a time when you will return phone messages—and you should mention it on your outgoing voice-mail message. Of course, you need times to do your work. You should consider being unavailable for calls or walk-ins (people who walk in to see you without calling first or having an appointment) during these times, especially if your time log shows that you are not completing work on time. On the other hand, you should also consider having times when walk-ins are welcome—true open-door times. Remember that time management does not mean scheduling work for yourself 24 hours a day. Set aside times for yourself; schedule lunch and even breaks if you must. Reserve time for family and vacations and stick to this schedule.

Not all tasks are created equal. Next, you will need to set priorities according to some system. Some people assign tasks priorities of 1, 2, 3, or A, B, C, or some other method.[70] The particulars are not as important as the act of prioritizing. Whatever method you use, you must separate tasks that must be performed immediately from those that can wait a while, that can wait a long time, and those that need to be given to others or don't need to be done at all. Once you establish broad categories and place tasks into them, you may have to go through each category and place those tasks in order.

The next question is, which item do you do first? Some people start at the top of their lists and simply work through the items. Others do the tasks they like first and the ones they don't like last. On the other hand, some reverse this, saving the jobs they like as a reward for completing the ones they dislike. Some people like to do all the little tasks first so that they see some progress; others want to dive right into the big job to get it behind them. Any of these methods can work as long as high-priority work is getting done, but if someone is using one of these methods to procrastinate and escape necessary work, then that person is wasting time, not managing it.

Time management isn't all about you however. Plenty of people in this world are perfectly happy to waste other people's time. Don't let them manage your time. Consider the following:

- Whenever possible go to other people's offices rather than having them come to you.[71] This way, you can leave when you are finished.
- Attend only those meetings that affect or interest you.[72] Few things are more frustrating than having work to do while stuck in a meeting that you don't need to be at.
- Set time limits for meetings and phone calls just as you would for any other task.[73] If you only have 5 minutes and some issue requires 25 minutes, then inform the person or persons and reschedule for when you do have time.
- Do not let people give you their emergencies. Failure to plan on their part does not constitute an emergency on yours.

Big Jobs

Throughout this discussion of managing time and tasks, prioritizing, and scheduling, it may have seemed as if all jobs were accomplished rather quickly and that the main problem is prioritizing and finding time to work. But what about the really big jobs? How does one even start a job that is too large to conceive of or to contemplate all at once? There are two keys to accomplishing large projects. There is a barrier you must first cross to complete a large project: it is called *starting*. Once you begin the project and have crossed this barrier, the project seems easier to handle. You may find that what is depressing is the thought of doing the project, not the actual performing of the activity. You must start any way you can. Even if it is only a small thing, you must start to be able to finish.

The second key is to divide the large, overwhelming project into a series of smaller easier-to-handle parts. Don't think of the entire project; think of the part you can complete this week, today, or by the end of this hour. If you limit your view to what you can accomplish during the current work session, then by constantly chipping away at the whole, you will eventually find yourself at the end of your large projects.

Summary

This chapter has explained management's responsibilities and the scope of management's job. The two main schools of management thought have been described along with the history of each. The two organizations existing in every workplace have been introduced along with your role as a managee in the organizations and in relation to

management. The goal of the chapter was to provide you with an understanding and appreciation of management's job.

In understanding work, management, and your relationship to each you should have observed a number of things. First, you should have observed the difference between your role as a managee and the role of your manager. You should have noted that managing is not easy, nor is it really an "advancement." Becoming a manager is really a career change. You should also have seen that duties in a modern organization are divided and that they are divided differently depending on whether you have a classical manager or situation or a behavioral manager or situation. In dividing these duties, this chapter has shown that some are the sole purview of the manager, whereas others are shared by the managers and managees.

You should be able to identify and classify the system you are working in and adapt to it. Just as a professional manager can adapt to the situation or the person, a professional employee can adapt to the situation or the manager. To be able to cope with and adapt to a given work situation not only increases your value to the employer, but reduces your stress and may increase your job satisfaction.

Self-management is growing in popularity, and according to some, virtually everyone in the future will be required to self-manage. Either with or without self-management, time-management skills will be needed. Time management not only aids in the accomplishment of routine tasks, but can be the key to working smarter, not harder.

REFERENCES

1. Daft, RL: Management, ed 5. Dryden, Fort Worth, 2000, p 37.
2. Pride, WM, et al: Business, ed 6. Houghton Mifflin, Boston, 1999, p 21.
3. Aldag, RJ, and Stearns, TM: Management, ed 2. Southwestern Publishing, Cincinnati, 1991, p 14.
4. Pride, et al, p 143.
5. Daft, pp 206–207.
6. Ibid, pp 146–147.
7. Scott, WR: Organizations: Rational, Natural, and Open Systems, ed 2. Prentice-Hall, Englewood Cliffs, NJ, 1987, p 5.
8. Aldag, RJ, and Stearns, TM, p 14.
9. Bateman, TS, and Zeithaml, CP: Management Function and Strategy, ed 2. Irwin, Homewood, Ill., 1993, p 413.
10. Veiga, JF, and Yanouzas, JN: The Dynamics of Organization Theory: Gaining a Macro Perspective, ed 2. West, St. Paul, 1984, p 258.
11. Boone, LE, and Bowen, DD, (eds): The Great Writings in Management and Organizational Behavior, ed 2. McGraw-Hill, New York, 1987, pp 34–52. Taylor, FW: The Principles of Scientific Management. Bulletin of the Taylor Society, December 1916, pp 13–23.
12. Daft, p 48.
13. Aldag, and Stearns, p 35.
14. Daft, p 49.

15. Weber, M: The Theory of Social and Economic Organization. Henderson, AM, and Parsons, T, trans. Free Press, New York, 1947, p 331.
16. Aldag, and Stearns, p 40.
17. Weber, pp 332–333.
18. Daft, p 46.
19. Scott, pp 31–35.
20. Higgins, JM: The Management Challenge. Macmillan, New York, 1991, p 36.
21. Tuchman, BW: A Distant Mirror. Ballantine, New York, 1978, p 5.
22. Boone, and Bowen, pp 34–36.
23. Burke, J: The Day the Universe Changed. Little, Brown & Company, Boston, 1985, pp 163–176.
24. Boone, and Bowen, pp 34–52.
25. Ibid, pp 50–52.
26. Van Fleet, DD: Contemporary Management, ed 2. Houghton Mifflin, Dallas, 1991, pp 40–45.
27. Daft, pp 47–49.
28. Aldag, and Stearns, p 48.
29. Daft, pp 49–50.
30. Higgins, p 45.
31. Hubbard, E: A Message To Garcia. Roycrafters, Aurora, New York, 1914.
32. Rue, LW, and Byars, LL: Management Theory and Application, ed 5. Irwin, Homewood, Ill., 1989, p 50.
33. Daft, pp 50–53.
34. Pride, et al, pp 277–78
35. Mayo, E: The Social Problems of an Industrial Civilization. Harvard College, Boston, 1945, pp 77–84.
36. Pride, et al, p 227.
37. Mayo, pp 69–76.
38. Higgins, p 5.
39. Rue, and Byars, p 47.
40. Daft, pp 540–42.
41. Stoner, JAF, and Freeman, RE: Management, ed 5. Prentice-Hall, Englewood Cliffs, NJ, 1992, pp 40–43.
42. Aldag, RJ, and Stearns, TM, pp 414–17.
43. Rue, LW, and Byars, LL, p 47.
44. Mondy, RW, et al: Management Concepts, Practices, and Skills, ed 5. Allyn and Bacon, Boston, 1991, pp 215–23.
45. Scott, pp 53–54.
46. Ibid, pp 54–56.
47. Mondy, et al, p 217.
48. Ibid, pp 219–20.
49. Boone, and Bowen, pp 38–39.
50. Mondy, et al, pp 221–22.
51. Collins, EGC, and Devanna, MA: The Portable MBA. John Wiley & Sons, New York, 1990, p 223.
52. Tyler, G: The Work Ethic: A Union View. It Comes with the Territory. Gini, AR, and Sullivan, TJ, eds. Random House, New York, 1989, p 128.
53. Andrew, J: DuBrin, Reengineering Survival Guide. Thomson Executive Press, Cincinnati, 1996, p 182.
54. Ivancevich, JM, et al: Management: Quality and Competitiveness. Irwin, Chicago, 1997, p 356.
55. Bensen, T: A brave new world? Industry Week, August 3, 1992:48–54.
56. Ivancevich, p 356.
57. Frayne, C, and Geringer, JM: Self-management training for joint venture general managers. Human Resource Planning, December 1992:75.
58. Ivancevich, p 356.
59. Ibid, pp 356–357. Frayne, C, and Geringer, JM, p 76.
60. Ibid, p 77.
61. McGarvey, R: More power to them. Entrepreneur, February 1995:74.
62. Holzman, D: When workers run the show. Working Woman, August 1993:73.
63. McGarvey, R, p 75.
64. Holzman, D, p 73.
65. Ibid, p 73.
66. Macan, TH: Time management. Test of a process Model. J Appl Psychol 79(3):381–391, 1994.
67. Lucco, FL: Effective time management. Appraisal, October 1994, p 582.
68. Paulson, TL: They Shoot Managers, Don't They? Ten Speed Press, Berkeley, Calif., 1991, p 49.
69. Alexander, R: Starving out the time gobblers. Superv Manage, February 1993, p 8.
70. Harris, L: Discipline your desk. Working Women, November 1994, p 8.
71. Alexander, R, p 8.
72. Brill, JE: Not enough hours. American Bar Association Journal, June 1992, p 98.
73. Ibid, p 98.

6 • The Informal Organization

Objectives

On completion of this chapter, the reader will be able to:

☐ Describe the informal organization.

☐ List and explain the reasons that people participate in informal organizations.

☐ Describe methods that may assist people in entering informal organizations and their groups.

☐ List and describe positive and negative contributions informal organizations can make in the working environment.

Chapter 5 introduced the working environment's formal and informal organizations. Both are critical to the functioning of any company. The formal organization is a deliberate management construct. It is typically described in writing, is codified in the operations of the organization, and is changed only after considerable contemplation. The informal organization is less rigid, more casual, and changes spontaneously. Because every member of the formal organization is also a member of, and is influenced by, the informal organization, this informal organization warrants additional scrutiny. Scrutiny of informal organizations cannot occur without some discussion of formal organizations, just as informal organizations themselves cannot exist without formal organizations.

The more specific an organization's rules of behavior are and the more the roles in the organization are separated from the people occupying those roles, the more formalized the organization is. Formalization also tries to make behavior more uniform, so it can be expected that people in similar positions will behave in similar ways. Formalization, then, is an attempt at making the organization more stable. It is also an attempt to make positions and relationships within the formal organization more apparent.[1] It is easier for people to identify their roles in an organization that is more formalized. However, there is still much that is unclear in even the most formal of organizations. This chapter will explore this ambiguity in addition to those areas in which organizations impact an employee's position.

What Is the Informal Organization?

In the previous chapter, the informal organization was introduced from a managerial point of view. This chapter will look at it from a managee's view. As mentioned in Chapter 5, the informal organization exists in conjunction with the formal organization. In an organization with a high degree of formalization, you will be able to discern your official role more readily. You will be able to see your position in the chain of command and read about it in a job description. However, as mentioned in Chapter 5, there probably will not be a contact chart describing the informal, or social, organization.[2] To understand this situation, the informal organization will be defined, and the reasons for group formation will be examined along with the reasons people enter groups. This should prepare you to break into the social network, and break in accurately describes the process.

Why People Join Informal Organization Groups

The informal organization is the set of unofficial relationships that develop between employees.[3] It is present in every organization, and it develops in addition to, and irrespective of, the formal organization. It is often ignored, its power is often underestimated, and it can be difficult for new employees to enter.[4] However, even though it is difficult to enter, virtually everyone tries to do so.

People join groups within the informal organization for these reasons:

- Social contacts
- Satisfaction of needs
- Power
- Peer pressure
- Help in solving work problems
- Goal congruency
- Understanding
- Information and communication
- Knowledge
- Formal organization support
- Physical proximity

Perhaps the biggest reason why people join informal organization groups is their need for *social contact*. Humans are social creatures. As such, they want to belong to and have contact with others. However, it is hard to feel a part of large organizations (and sometimes those not so large). So people form smaller, more easily identifiable and comprehensible groups. In fact, it is almost required. Fifty percent of the employees that quit their jobs do so in the first 6 months. A prime reason for leaving is that social contacts were not made.[5]

People join groups to *satisfy needs* for belonging (as just mentioned) and for status and self-esteem. People who lack an official position with sufficient status to suit them may work at leading a group of peers. If they do not get status (and self-esteem) from their job, they may substitute the status received from peers (and therefore derive self-esteem). These people may lead the group with, or against, the formal organization and the organization's goals.[6] In health care a serious side effect to some informal organization actions is less than desirable patient care. A professional employee would not participate in informal organization activities that may be harmful to patients or clients.

The old saying that "there is strength in numbers" explains another aspect of why people join groups. The *power* of a group increases that of an individual. This enables the individual, the group, or both to better accomplish their goals.[7]

Another reason you may join a particular work clique is sometimes related to the "power in numbers" idea. You may join a group because of *peer pressure*. Because people believe there is power in numbers, when you are new to a job, various cliques may try to recruit you. Some may wait awhile to "size you up" (to see what your values are). However, some may start right from the beginning to bring you in on their side. Not only can the pressure to join a group be strong, but the groups can have a very effective weapon against you if you try to resist. Failure to join either a group or the group recruiting you can lead to *ostracism*. Because humans are social creatures and because most people seek some degree of social contact at work, being ostracized or isolated from others can be an effective punishment or a strong inducement to join a group, or both.

Joining a group can *help in solving problems*. Whether work related or not, it is often easier to talk about problems with members of a peer group. In work situations, many people are more comfortable with getting help from coworkers than managers. Many people do not want to appear unknowledgeable in front of the person who evaluates them.[8]

Some people join informal organization groups because of *goal congruency*—that is, the goals of the

 Building Comprehension Exercise begins on following page

BUILDING COMPREHENSION EXERCISE 6–1

Evaluating Informal Organization Factors

Define each of the following components of the informal organization in your words. Then rank the importance to you of each from 1 to 11, with 1 being most important. Why are the top five important to you?

Rank

____ Social contacts

_____

_____

_____ Satisfaction of needs

_____

_____

____ Power

_____

_____

____ Peer pressure

_____

_____

____ Help in solving work problems

_____

_____

____ Goal congruency

_____

_____

____ Understanding

_____

_____

Exercise continues on following page

_____ Information and communication

_____

_____

_____ Knowledge

_____

_____

_____ Formal organization support

_____

_____

_____ Physical proximity

_____

_____

End of exercise. Text continues on following page.

group match those of the individual.[9] These goals may be inside or outside the context of work. Sometimes people band together because the changes they wish to make in working conditions are the same. Other times the common goal may be outside of work, as when members of the same volunteer organization or amateur athletic team stay together as a group during work hours.

People enter groups because they share goals, as just discussed, and because they share experiences. They seek *understanding* from people who know well the trials and tribulations of the job. Friends outside of work and family members may lend a sympathetic ear, but unless they have been through similar situations, it may not be meaningful. This may be especially true in the health-care fields. Many health professions are highly stressful and demanding, even those that do not center on life-or-death care. It seems to help to talk about these things with others who have been there.

Still another reason you may ally yourself with a particular group or make certain informal connections is to receive *information*. The informal communication chain is commonly referred to as the *grapevine*, and it often transmits information much faster than the official lines.[10] However, it can transmit misinformation with equal speed. You must be careful about how you use grapevine information and to whom you pass it on.

People sometimes look to a group for *protection*. They may seek protection from a manager, "the system," or the pressures of the job. The last reason is similar to one of the reasons given when *understanding* was discussed.

You may also turn to a group or an individual other than your manager when you have a work problem because the group members have the experience and education to help you. *Knowledge* is one of the most respected things a coworker can possess. People will go to the person who knows the most about the job, even if that person does not hold an official position. It is also possible for people to come together for advice and support, thus forming a group for information sharing.

The informal organization may *support the formal organization*.[11] Shortcomings, power vacuums, inadequacies, and a temporary crisis in the formal structure can all be fulfilled by the informal organization. The informal leadership and groups can sometimes be the main reason the department or organization functions. The spectrum or compensating behavior that can be found in informal organizations can range from getting by when the manager is sick or on vacation to providing support without which a collapse of the organization would result.[12]

The final impetus for informal group formation

on this list is *physical proximity*. People who work together have a greater tendency to form an informal work group. Obviously, if people do not have opportunities for contact, it will be difficult, if not impossible, for them to form an identifiable group.[13]

Joining Informal Organization Groups

Almost everyone will enter the informal organization or some group within it for the reasons just described. Most do so in a haphazard way. But, there are behaviors you can exhibit that may speed your entry into the social structure of the working environment.[14]

JOB KNOWLEDGE

Probably the one attribute that coworkers respect most is job knowledge. However, especially in the beginning, such knowledge must be revealed delicately. Flaunting your job knowledge, being arrogant, or using it to make others feel foolish or to embarrass them is *not* the best way to make new friends. Historically, we in the United States expect our heroes, and our superiors, to be good but humble. We do not suffer braggarts. Use your job knowledge to do your job well and to give helpful suggestions to others. Until you know people better, it is wiser to suggest alternatives than to state solutions (and if you are not sure about something, then you can follow my father's advice, "It is better to remain silent and be thought a fool, than to open your mouth and remove all doubt").

WORK PERFORMANCE

Doing your share of the workload is almost always a good way to be appreciated by the boss *and* accepted by your peers. Be available where the work is. Do *not* camp out in the lounge. Do *not* be a clock watcher. Do *not* take breaks longer than specified. Arrive on time. Perform your work quickly while still delivering quality patient care. It may even be acceptable to do a little more than others, but here can arise a dilemma. Managers want people to work as fast and hard as possible. On the other hand, the informal organization may exert pressure on people to conform to the group's rate. *Rate busters* are people who exceed a group's standards, and they are not appreciated. The fear is that the manager may discover that a higher rate is possible,

 Building Comprehension Exercise begins on following page

BUILDING COMPREHENSION EXERCISE 6–2

Joining Informal Groups

Define and rate yourself on each of the behaviors related to joining informal groups.

Job Knowledge

Definition _____

Rating:

____ A. I am one of the most knowledgeable people in my field.

____ B. I possess above average knowledge in my field.

____ C. I possess average knowledge in my field.

____ D. I possess less than average knowledge in my field.

____ E. I am one of the least knowledgeable people in my field.

Work Performance

Definition _____

Rating:

____ A. I typically do much more work than my coworkers.

____ B. I typically do somewhat more work than my coworkers.

____ C. I typically do the same amount of work as my coworkers.

____ D. I typically do somewhat less work than my coworkers.

____ F. I typically do much less work than my coworkers.

Exercise continues on following page 🎁🎁🎁

Dependability

Definition _____

Rating:

_____ A. I never miss a day of work.

_____ B. I rarely miss work.

_____ C. I sometimes miss work.

_____ D. I miss at least 6 days of work per year.

_____ E. I typically miss 1 day of work per month.

_____ A. I arrive at work at least a few minutes early virtually every day.

_____ B. I arrive at work on time virtually every day.

_____ C. I arrive at work on time most days.

_____ D. I arrive at work late about 1 day per month.

_____ E. I arrive at work late 1 or more days per week.

_____ A. I complete almost all work tasks in less time than expected.

_____ B. I complete most work tasks in less time than expected.

_____ C. I complete almost all work tasks on time.

_____ D. I complete some work tasks in more time than expected.

_____ E. I complete almost all work tasks in more time than expected.

Willingness to Help Others

Definition _____

Rating:

_____ A. I always assist my coworkers whenever they ask me to.

_____ B. I assist my coworkers more than others do.

_____ C. I assist my coworkers about as much as others do.

_____ D. I rarely assist my coworkers.

_____ E. I never assist my coworkers.

Exercise continues on following page 🔲🔲🔲

Challenging Group Norms

Definition _____

Rating:

_____ A. I never challenge the group norms.

_____ B. I rarely challenge the group norms.

_____ C. I only occasionally challenge the group norms.

_____ D. I sometimes challenge the group norms.

_____ E. I routinely challenge the group norms.

Ask, Don't Tell

Definition _____

Rating: If I were a new employee and I saw someone do something that I thought was wrong, I would

_____ A Ask them why they are doing it that way.

_____ B. Not say anything.

_____ C. Ask if they have ever done it another way.

_____ D. Ask them why they are doing it wrong.

_____ E. Tell them they are doing it wrong.

Socialize

Definition _____

Rating: When I find myself with people I do not know, I

_____ A. Start conversations with others.

_____ B. Answer questions with details, and then ask others about themselves.

_____ C. Answer only the question I am asked.

_____ D. Interrupt others with stories of myself.

_____ E. Say nothing, even when asked.

Exercise continues on following page 🎲 🎲 🎲

Review your answers, writing 4 in front of every "A" you checked off, 3 in front of every "B" you checked, 2 for every "C," 1 for every "D," and 0 for every "E." Total your score. If you scored between 36 and 27, you should have few problems, if any, fitting into the informal organization. If you scored between 26 and 18, it may take a little longer, but you should eventually fit in with the informal organization. Working on any areas where you checked answers "D" or "E" could help. If you scored between 17 and 9, it may take much longer for you to fit into the informal organization, and you should consider working on areas where you checked answers "D" or "E." If you scored 8 or less, you will probably have significant difficulty fitting into the informal organization. You should work hard to change every area where you answered "C," "D," and "E."

End of exercise. Text continues on following page.

and that rate will come to be expected. This concern is certainly valid because managers have taken such action in industry throughout history.

DEPENDABILITY

Managers and informal organization group members appreciate dependability in their coworkers. Reliable coworkers are on the job at the right time, present every day, and able to carry out a task at a level that is acceptable or better with relatively little supervision or direction. In other words, be known as a person who can be counted on to do the job correctly the first time.

WILLINGNESS TO HELP OTHERS

Social groups also look at your willingness to help others. This does not mean doing their work for them. Instead, it means assisting people with tasks requiring more than one person. Lifting patients is a good example. Volunteer to help—offer, rather than wait to be asked. This help will be reciprocated later when you need some assistance.

CHALLENGING GROUP NORMS

Do not challenge group norms. All groups have behaviors or rules that members are expected to observe. Challenging the rules is not popular when you belong to the group. Defying or ignoring them is even less well-tolerated when you have yet to be accepted by the group. Going along with the group standards will speed your acceptance by the existing members and is permissible if the standards do not violate ethical, legal, organizational, and, of course, patient care standards. For example, in some workplaces it is customary for people to bring cake or donuts for everyone on their birthday. Conforming to this simple group norm demonstrates a willingness to belong to the group.

ASK, DON'T TELL

People who have worked somewhere longer than you have (which is just about everyone when you first start out) do not appreciate being told what to do. This is especially true when you are right and they are wrong. If you tell them they are wrong, but it is really you who is wrong, they can forgive your ignorance—after all, you're new. If you are *right*, they may resent you for a long, long

time. If you think someone is doing something wrong, it is better to ask him or her about it than to command the person to change. Say something like, "Isn't this usually done this way?" If the coworker has a good reason for doing this thing differently, then you will not look so foolish. If he or she does not have a reason, if he or she is wrong, the mistake can be corrected with a minimum of embarrassment.

SOCIALIZE

A good way to be accepted into a work group or department is to get to know people. Introduce yourself, go on break and to lunch with different people, share training and work experiences, and discuss your life outside of work—in other words, get to know them and let them get to know you. Most people form groups with people who are like themselves. They have the same values, come from similar backgrounds, and so on. Just making the effort to know, and be known by, your coworkers will go a long way toward helping you break into the social environment.

Summary

It is doubtful that any formal organization could be created to account for all contingencies.[15] Possibly the most significant benefit of informal organizations is their ability to answer needs unmet by the formal organization. This, and the numerous social needs of people, explains the existence of informal organizations.

The informal, or social, organization exists in every work environment with more than one person in it. Social contacts are one of the reasons people work. The informal organization is powerful. It can affect you in positive or negative ways, and breaking into it is difficult. This chapter has outlined the reasons people join these groups and ways to assist you in joining them. The increased awareness of these informal organization characteristics should help you to cope with them and the people in them.

REFERENCES

1. Scott, WR: Organizations: Rational, Natural and Open Systems, ed 2. Prentice-Hall, Englewood Cliffs, NJ, 1987, p 33.
2. Phillips, RI: The informal organization in your hospital. Radiol Technol 46:2, 1974.
3. Mondy, RW, et al: Management: Concepts, Practices, and Skills. Allyn and Bacon, Boston, 1991, p 215.

4. Smith, HC, and Wakeley, JH: Psychology of Industrial Behavior, ed 3. McGraw-Hill, New York, 1972, p 7.
5. Mondy, et al, p 220.
6. Aldag, RJ, and Stearns, TM: Management. Southwestern Publishing, Cincinnati, 1991, p 537.
7. Ibid, p 537.
8. Mondy, et al, p 220.
9. Aldag, and Stearns, p 537.
10. Mondy, et al, p 220.
11. Phillips, p 101.
12. Mondy, et al, p 220.
13. Aldag, and Stearns, p 535.
14. Ibid, pp 540–41.
15. Phillips, p 104.

7 ∘ Performance Evaluations

Objectives

On completion of this chapter, the reader will be able to:

☐ List and describe the stated and unstated criteria managers often use to evaluate managees.

☐ Identify biases that raters may possess.

☐ Describe possible responses to specific rater biases.

☐ Describe possible responses to substandard evaluations.

☐ Describe risks associated with challenging an evaluation.

☐ Describe recommendations for presenting evaluation challenges.

Ideally, performance evaluations should not only be a review of past performance, they should also be a tool for helping improve future performance. To perform well and receive a good evaluation, you must begin by knowing the criteria that will be used in judging you. The best time to ask to see a blank evaluation is during the interview for the job. Reading the job description for the position you are interviewing for may seem adequate, because the performance evaluation should arise from the job description. This is not always the case. The performance evaluation is what will be used to rate you, and the quality of the evaluation may reveal something of the caliber of the prospective employer. Reviewing the performance evaluation will assist you in deciding on whether or not to take the position, and you will know exactly what the job entails and what is expected of you right from the start.

You may need to proceed differently if the prospective employer does not have a written performance evaluation. This may be true of those employing a small number of people. In this case it is still a good idea to ask during the job interview how you will be judged. It will be less awkward for you to ask about the evaluation process at this time than after you have accepted the position. The worst time to discover what the performance standards are is during the evaluation. To further ensure that you are fully informed when you are evaluated, you should know about the challenges the evaluation process presents.

Common Criteria

You should be aware of hidden, unmentioned performance standards and other problems and challenges of evaluations. The following criteria may or may not be stated, but they are important to almost every manager. They are:

- Dependability
- Job knowledge
- Organization
- Efficiency
- Interacting with people
- Attitude

Managers consistently rate dependability near the top of their list of items influencing their evaluations. Many prefer an average employee who is dependable over a better performer who is unreliable. In other words, it doesn't matter how good you are if you are not there.

Job knowledge is important for obvious reasons. The more you know, the more valuable you are to your employer. Job knowledge also earns the most respect from coworkers.

Organization and efficiency are closely related. It is possible to be highly organized and not efficient—spending a lot of time organizing can slow some people down. On the other hand, it is hard to be efficient when one is not organized. Both can influence your score on other areas and both are common criteria themselves.

Interacting with people is especially important in health care, whether the people are patients, clients, coworkers, or managers. Your dealings with them influence your evaluation even if this is not explicitly stated.

Attitude is a nebulous criterion. It can also be second only to dependability for some bosses. Managers and coworkers want someone who is cooperative, agreeable, understanding, and supportive.

Preparing for an Evaluation

Evaluations should review your past performance, establish your current position, and examine future intentions. To ensure that you and your manager maximize the value of an evaluation, you should both prepare for it. Too often, employees stand in judgment before the manager. Sometimes this is true because the manager has been forced into this position. The manager must evaluate the managees. If the managees have nothing to say, then the burden falls on the manager. The manager may review the past, but it is difficult to plan a managee's future without his or her help. So the evaluation degrades into a situation where the manager reviews what he or she has seen and passes judgment, and the ordeal is over until next year. An evaluation does not have to be this way. If you become involved in your evaluation by preparing for it, evaluations can be an important method of professional advancement.

Becoming involved in your evaluation by preparing for it means that you follow the guidelines for a good evaluation. You review what you have done in the past, you examine your current status, and you plan for the future. Evaluating yourself and doing it objectively is not easy, but if you want to be a professional, you must advance, and this procedure is all but required to advance.

In examining the past, you should evaluate what you have done since your last evaluation. Identify areas where you have improved as well as areas that need further improvement. When first reviewing your performance, resist the urge to rationalize poor performance. List all of the significant things you did. Once this is done, you can review the reasons behind your performance. When looking for the reasons for poor performance, you must avoid blaming others. It is difficult to admit that some poor performance was solely your fault, but this is necessary if you are to improve. It is not necessarily bad to make mistakes; it is bad not to learn from mistakes. To learn from mistakes, you must examine the cause, analyze what went wrong, and change your behavior in the future.

In examining your current status, you may consider three perspectives. You may wish to examine where you are now in relation to your career, employment, and last evaluation. Some of this information may be only for your benefit, but it is important to periodically examine your career, and your evaluation is a good time to do that. Your manager may be most concerned with your status in relation to your last evaluation, but it is often in your best interest to show how far you have come since you were hired.

Planning for the future can be the most valuable portion of an evaluation. The past is over; what was done is done. The future allows for growth and improvement. *Growth* refers to areas in which you perform well, or not at all, but wish to expand to. *Improvement* refers to tasks you currently perform but do not perform well. Ensure that both growth and improvement, and not just improvement, are reviewed during the evaluation.

To receive the maximum benefit from the planning process, you should review your previous goals, identify those that you met and those that you did not, and identify those you want to carry into the next evaluation period. After reviewing previous goals, you may create new ones. Some people set a goal of changing job responsibilities or earning a promotion. Setting a goal well in advance leads to an important evaluation question.

If you have as a goal obtaining a promotion or a transfer or assuming additional duties, then there is an important question to be asked during your evaluation. Before actually applying for a promotion, you should ask your manager, "If I applied for that position today, is there anything that would keep me from getting it?" Asking this will help you identify areas to work on. These areas can then be included in your plans for the future. For example, assume you wish to become a supervisor next year. On asking your manager if there is anything that would keep you from becoming a supervisor, she replies, "Yes. You know the job and the department well, but you really need to complete a Principles of Management course." Now you know what needs to be done to obtain your future goal of becoming a supervisor—you must set a more immediate goal of completing a course in management.

A further benefit of preparing for an interview is that you demonstrate that you are enthusiastic, concerned, and involved with your work and your profession. The preparation will reflect positively on you and will probably result in higher evaluation scores. Even though you prepare for an interview, there is no guarantee that it will go well because your being prepared doesn't mean your manager will be. Prepared or not, you may have an inaccurate or unfair evaluation to which you feel compelled to respond. Responses to evaluations require careful consideration, however, and they will be discussed further in this chapter.

Evaluator Bias

The criteria described previously may or may not be stated on the evaluation form (Fig. 7–1). When they are not, it has been shown that they still affect a manager's rating of an employee. Other concerns may arise because most managers and managees are uncomfortable with evaluations. Some concerns are caused by a lack of rater training. Managees should be aware of these to avoid unfair and inaccurate ratings. The additional factors that may consciously or subconsciously bias a rater's judgment include:

- Vague terms
- Insufficient data
- Different standards
- Extreme leniency
- Everyone-is-average personal philosophy
- Extreme strictness
- Leniency to avoid conflicts
- The halo effect
- Job importance
- Recent events
- Measuring of traits, not performance
- The rater's personal bias
- Deliberate downgrading

Before continuing, complete Building Comprehension Exercise 7–1.

Your performance is "poor," "bad," or "needs help." You miss work "frequently"; you are late

"often." Evaluations that use *vague terms* are not very informative and make the measurement of future performance difficult. How do you correct "poorness"? How many times constitutes "frequently" or "often"? If "poorness" is not defined, how will you know if you are getting better or poorer? If these kinds of words are used, ask the rater to be specific. Ask for the number of workdays you missed or the number of times you were late. When the manager says, "Your reject rate is 15 percent, whereas the department average is 6 percent and the range is 4 to 16 percent," he or she has said something concrete. Being specific not only identifies the problem but also allows the manager and employee to set future goals in terms that can be measured.[1]

The problem of *insufficient data* occurs when the rater is too far removed from the situation to form an accurate opinion. Your direct supervisor should make all evaluations. Anyone else is probably not familiar enough with your work to give it an accurate appraisal. Another manager may have an opinion about your performance, but it will be based only on a few encounters or on information filtered through others, or both.[2]

Each manager has *different standards*. Therefore, there will be variations in each one's ratings based on areas each feels is most important, each person's perceptions, or each rater's point of view. For example, as mentioned in the chapter on communications (see Chap. 3), people tend to give a higher rating to people they like, are extroverted, and are similar to themselves. Or, if your manager feels punctuality is vital, those who are on time or early may get higher ratings than others despite the job performance of each. Sometimes you can find out which areas are important to a manager just by openly asking him or her. Other times you may have to find out through the informal organization. In either case it is as important to know a manager's attitudes and feelings as it is to know the formal criteria on the performance evaluation.[3]

Extreme leniency in performance appraisals occurs when the rater gives everyone high marks.[4] Although this may not seem to harm you, it is actually doing you a disservice. As mentioned previously, performance evaluations should be used to measure past performance and to assist in improving future performance. This can come from correcting weak areas or from giving you opportunities to add skills. When everyone receives high marks, the upper-level managers will know the evaluations are worthless. Those truly deserving high evaluations will not stand out and may not receive advanced opportunities. Also, when word gets around that everyone received the same marks, the evaluation will become a disincentive.

Identifies self and position to patients, families, and visitors whenever working with them by wearing name badge and verbally introducing self, using first name, and stating job title
Excellent performance: 100% of the time
Acceptable performance: 99.9–98% of the time
Poor performance: 97.9–93% of the time
Unacceptable performance: Less than 92.9% of the time

Arrives to work at the assigned starting time
Excellent performance: Arrives on time every day
Acceptable performance: Is late by no more than 7 minutes,1 or 2 day per month
Poor performance: Is late by no more than 7 minutes, 3 to 5 days per month
Unacceptable performance: Is late 6 or more days per month

Performs examinations within plus or minus 10% of the time allotted for the type of exam
Excellent performance: 100% of the time
Acceptable performance: 99.9–90% of the time
Poor performance: 89.9–75% of the time
Unacceptable performance: Less than 74.9% of the time

Conducts procedures according to established procedures
Excellent performance: 100% of the time
Acceptable performance: 99.9–97% of the time
Poor performance: 96.9–93% of the time
Unacceptable performance: Less than 92.9% of the time

Arranges equipment for examinations
Excellent performance: 100% of the time
Acceptable performance: 99.9–95% of the time
Poor performance: 94.9–90% of the time
Unacceptable performance: Less than 89.9% of the time

Confirms identity of patient scheduled for an exam with 100% accuracy
Excellent performance: All patients correctly identified
Poor performance: Exam performed on wrong patient once
Unacceptable performance: Exam performed on wrong patient twice

Increases knowledge by participating in monthly department meetings
Excellent performance: Attends 12 meetings per year
Acceptable performance: Attends 11 to 9 meetings per year
Poor performance: Attends 8 to 6 meetings per year
Unacceptable performance: Attends 5 or fewer meetings per year

Reports equipment malfunctions
Excellent performance: Within 5 minutes of each malfunction
Acceptable performance: Within 6 to 15 minutes of each malfunction
Poor performance: Within 15 to 30 minutes of each malfunction
Unacceptable performance: Takes 31 or more minutes

FIGURE 7–1 • Sample performance appraisal items. Notice that these items are clear, objective, and measurable.

Why work harder if you can do less and still get the same rating as everyone else?

A similar disincentive materializes when *everyone is graded as average*. This practice has the same effect as giving everyone high marks; it shows there is no reason to be more productive.[5]

Another problem that can arise from everyone having been rated high or average can occur when a new manager takes over. The new person may be expecting adequate or superior performance based on previous ratings. If accurate ratings are not available, the manager may give lower ratings, maybe lower than deserved. The cause may be that the difference between the old evaluations and new is greater than the new manager expected because the old evaluations are artificially high or at least higher than deserved.

Just as some managers are overly lenient, others are prone to *extreme strictness*.[6] However, like extreme leniency, strictness is not only a disincentive,

 Building Comprehension Exercise begins on following page

Recognizing Evaluator Bias

Before reading the definitions in the text, try to define each of these examples of evaluator bias. Then try to predict the effect each of these would have on workers.

Vague terms

Definition: _____

_____

Effect on workers: _____

_____

Insufficient data

Definition: _____

_____

Effect on workers: _____

_____

Different standards

Definition: _____

_____

Effect on workers: _____

_____

Extreme leniency

Definition: _____

_____

Effect on workers: _____

_____

Exercise continues on following page 🔲 🔲 🔲

Everyone-is-average personal philosophy

Definition: _____

_____

Effect on workers: _____

_____

Extreme strictness

Definition: _____

_____

Effect on workers: _____

_____

Leniency to avoid conflicts

Definition: _____

_____

Effect on workers: _____

_____

The halo effect

Definition: _____

_____

Effect on workers: _____

_____

Job importance

Definition: _____

_____

Effect on workers: _____

_____

Exercise continues on following page 🔳🔳🔳

Recent events

Definition: _____

_____

Effect on workers: _____

_____

Measuring of traits, not performance

Definition: _____

_____

Effect on workers: _____

_____

The rater's personal bias

Definition: _____

_____

Effect on workers: _____

_____

Deliberate downgrading

Definition: _____

_____

Effect on workers: _____

_____

End of exercise. Text continues on following page.

it is also demoralizing. To be rated lower than your performance level can decrease your feelings of self-esteem and self-worth.

Some managers practice *leniency to avoid conflicts.* They give people ratings that they feel will appease or placate them; thus, they avoid having to discuss poor performance with anyone. Although such leniency may allow managers to avoid manager-managee confrontations, it is yet another disincentive for people to work hard, and it does them a disservice by not helping them to improve.

The *halo effect* is another rater error, but one that few employees would complain about. It occurs usually when the rater allows one outstanding characteristic to influence the rating of other criteria.[7] Accordingly, a person with a high quantity of output might receive a high rating for quality, whether it is deserved or not. The halo effect can also occur when a person has received past evaluations that are high. Some raters will not check closely on the period in question. They just assume that the past good performance is continuing. You may not consider the halo effect unfair when it is applied to you, but you might if it is applied to others and not to you.

One of Max Weber's principles of organization theory (the separation principle discussed in Chap. 5) states that the position must be separate from the person occupying the position. Thus, there are job evaluations to examine positions in a company and performance evaluations to appraise the people in those positions. Commonly, *job importance* affects a person's review.[8] The result is that people in higher positions receive higher performance evaluations because of the position they occupy and possibly not because they deserve them.

Being judged on *recent events* can work for you or against you. This judgment involves the rater's giving more weight to your performance during the period just before your evaluation than to the rest of the evaluation period.[9] If you receive annual evaluations and you performed adequately for most of the year but the week or two before your evaluation things went bad for you, then recent events could work against you. If most of the year was bad for you but the month before your evaluation the situation improved, then recent events could work in your favor. Of course, not all raters fall victim to this error, and some of those who do, do so somewhat innocently. What can happen is that a manager may receive a notice from the human resources (personnel) department that you are due for an annual review. Usually this comes 2 to 4 weeks before your anniversary date. The manager then realizes it is time to pay some

attention to what you have been doing. On the other hand, some employees (and students) count on recent-events error—they only put forth their best effort just before their review (or, in the case of students, just before they graduate). You should be aware that many managers (maybe even the majority) have good memories when it comes to remembering poor work, tardiness, and so on; they may not be so easily fooled.

Sometimes the evaluation process *measures traits and not performance.* Here, your personality is evaluated more than your performance.[10,11] For example, an extrovert with average performance may receive a higher rating than an introvert with above-average performance. A top performer with an "attitude problem" may get a lower score than a "company person" who is mediocre. Performance should be based on objective, measurable criteria that are related to the job, not to personality traits that do not have an impact on job performance.

A rater's *personal bias* may enter into the performance evaluation, helping some and hurting others. People tend to rate people who are like themselves and attractive higher than others. This bias can be based on sex, race, color, religion, age, politics, sports interests, willingness to contribute to the rater's favorite charity, and many other factors.[12] Having the evaluation based on objective, measurable criteria related to the job (as just mentioned) can work toward preventing this. Also, some evaluations require the rater to explain less-than-average scores. If yours does not, it behooves you to request them, preferably in writing. If the low ratings are justified, the manager should not object to writing out the reasons for them.

The final rating error is also the most insidious. *Deliberate downgrading* involves purposely giving someone a lower rating than he or she deserves. Sometimes the manager wants to decrease your chances for promotion (and maybe make someone else look better), or he or she may be trying to get you fired or justify not giving all or a large part of a merit raise. There are even some managers that do it in a misguided attempt to motivate people. They believe a lower rating will make people work harder to get a better rating next time.

One health-care manager that I knew of had a system for deliberately downgrading people with merit pay to lower her budget. This particular hospital usually gave everyone a 2 percent raise, with an additional 1 to 5 percent available based on merit. This manager would start severely criticizing people about 1 month before their annual review date. By the review date, an outsider would have thought the person was sure to be fired. Instead, the manager would review the "terrible"

 Building Comprehension Exercise begins on following page

BUILDING COMPREHENSION EXERCISE 7–2

Responding to an Evaluation

Amelia is your supervisor. In the last few years she has been assigned more and more managed-care paperwork to handle. As a result, she is not around much. In fact, she is so pressed for time that her manager, Janelle, conducted your annual performance review 6 weeks ago. Before that you only saw Janelle twice, and that was in the 2 weeks just before your review. Before that, you weren't really sure what she looked like. During the evaluation she said things like, "I would like you to try harder" and "I think you need to do better." She also said that she had heard you had been late returning from lunch and breaks a few times. Still, she said that she would give you about the same ratings she gave everyone else this year. She had little choice, she said, because there was no money for any merit increases (normally another 2 to 5.5 percent above the cost-of-living increase that everyone receives), and any "excellent" ratings would warrant an increase according to company policies. She also said that she would try to put all this in writing, but it has been 6 weeks, and you have seen nothing yet.

First, identify any evaluator biases you feel are present here. Write out the sentence from the scenario that supports your claim that a particular bias is present.

Bias	*Supporting Evidence*

Second, determine how you should respond, and why you should or should not respond. Create a detailed plan of what you will do. You think you have had one of your better years because your productivity increased 12.37 percent.

_____

_____

_____

_____

_____

End of exercise. Text continues on following page.

performances and then pretend to be doing them a favor by giving 2 percent for merit pay when supposedly none was deserved. She kept her budget lower, and she thought she came out looking like a good person for "giving" people at least a little something when they really didn't deserve it. She would then spend the next month pointing out only the good things each postreview person did. This step was to keep them from quitting after the evaluation ordeal and to give her the opportunity to point out the "improvements" her methods had wrought. In fact, very little changed. Veterans made a joke of the "bad month." ("My evaluation must be coming up; she's on my back constantly lately!") The most amazing thing is that people generally stayed, and no one challenged her. It is possible that no one challenged her because no one knew what responses were possible.

Possible Responses

Of course, only those evaluations that you feel are inaccurate require a response. Notice that I said *inaccurate*; I did not say that *negative* evaluations require a response. It is difficult to cope with receiving a negative evaluation. It is possible that it is inaccurate, but it is also possible that it is accurate and that someone is reluctant to accept it as true. No one wants to be told or to admit that they are not doing well. If a manager finds fault with your performance, you should carefully consider your response, which can often be difficult (Figs. 7–2 and 7–3). First, try to objectively evaluate the evaluation. Ask yourself, "Is it true and accurate?" If it is, you must then try to analyze why this has happened. Is it lack of experience? Lack of knowledge? Lack of training? Poor communications? Did you misinterpret what the job entailed? Did you not know what criteria the manager felt were most important? Are you just not very good at this job? Were there problems in your personal life? It is most important for you to be honest with yourself. When you have discovered why you were accurately rated low, you will be ready for the next difficult step.

Once you know why you have been doing poorly, you can look for ways to improve. Find out what is wrong, and then find out how to correct it. Maybe you need:

- More employer training
- More experience with a certain situation
- More supervision
- More studying and practice on your own

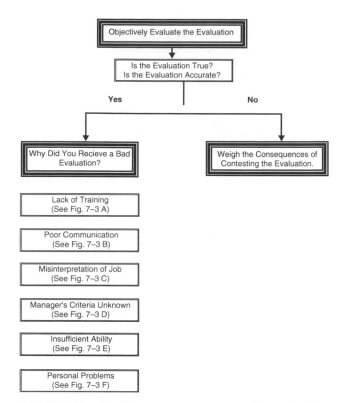

FIGURE 7–2 • Possible responses to a negative evaluation.

- A college course
- More time to perform certain tasks

Or perhaps you need something else. If your evaluator or boss has not recommended one or more of these to you, then you should suggest them. This will usually impress your boss because many people would not show this kind of motivation and concern to improve.

The last thing to do in the face of a poor performance rating is to learn from it and work hard at trying to improve. The world has plenty of people willing to do their jobs at the lowest acceptable level (and many more not even willing to do that). If you aspire to become a professional, especially a health-care professional, then you will take it upon yourself to do the best job you can (and not the least that can be gotten away with).

If you truly believe you have been judged unfairly, you have two major decisions to make. First, whether or not to respond, and second, how to respond. Both of these require that you to know the political environment at work if you are to minimize the risks you are taking.

There are always risks involved when challenging a manager. You are the only one who can decide whether or not a challenge is worth the risk. Appraise the situation, and make a list of things you stand to gain and those you may lose in disputing the evaluation. Some of the questions you

Cause of Negative Evaluation	Possible Actions
A Lack of Training	Request more training from your employer. Seek additional education on your own.
B Poor Communication	Prepare a list of questions and concerns; meet and discuss these with your *supervisor/manager*.
C Misinterpretation of Job	Clarify the exact nature of the duties, responsibilities, working conditions, and equipment required for your job. Ask for an updated copy of your job description or ask for similar information in writing.
D Manager's Criteria Unknown	Meet with your supervisor/manager and request a written copy of the performance appraisal (or other list) containing all criteria used to determine if your job is being adequately performed. Ask your supervisor/manager to specifically state what evidence is used to determine adequate performance.
E Insufficient Ability	Improve skills through education and practice. Consider a related career. Consider a different career.
F Personal Problems	Resolve problems. Meet with your manager to explain past problems, outline solutions, and commit to better performance in the future.

FIGURE 7–3 • Possible actions that you could take after receiving an accurate negative evaluation. (Consult after reviewing Fig. 7–2.)

should ask yourself while you are examining the situation are:

- Are evaluations ever used for anything here, or are they filed away, never to be looked at again?
- How have others fared when they challenged an evaluation?
- Were any of those situations like mine?
- Am I going to be here long enough for a bad evaluation to affect me?
- Is this just a matter of pride or hurt feelings, or are there real issues at stake here?
- How much support does your evaluator have from his or her managers?

Compare the possible gains to the possible losses. For example, do people who protest their evaluations get punished in some form later, are they labeled as troublemakers, and so on. The conservative approach would be to look at the lowest possible gain (which is often nothing) and the greatest possible loss. If the loss outweighs the gain, then it may not be a good idea to pursue a formal challenge or response.

It is not my intention to dissuade anyone from protesting an injustice; however, just because you are right does not mean you will win or gain. I want you to know that this is an imperfect world and that this is an uphill battle. Organizational politics may be at work, and they can be very powerful. Even if there is no political agenda, the status accorded evaluators will put them somewhat ahead from the beginning in almost all institutions—even those that have formal response mechanisms. If you do decide to continue with a response, there are some recommendations you can follow.

In contesting an evaluation, you generally have two initial paths to follow—the formal and the informal. The informal approach involves your meeting with the rater privately, but at lunch or on break, without an appointment. Here you would probably lodge a mild protest, something like, "I've given more thought to my evaluation, and I think that . . . ." Then you would mention the area of contention, usually without mentioning any specific redress or at most saying, "Could you review the situation again, and let me know if there is any change?" This may change nothing, and the only accomplishment may be to let the evaluator know that you disagreed. Or he or she may review the rating and make a change. In either case, this is relatively nonthreatening for the evaluator and usually less risky for you.

A formal protest may proceed in three ways: through the evaluator, through the evaluator's manager, or through the human resources (personnel) department. Organization policy or the lack of a human resources department may dictate which way to go. Otherwise, it is usually best to start with the evaluator. This is what following the chain of command is all about. Many times the boss's boss will insist you discuss the matter with your boss first. It is good conflict management and common courtesy to start with the person you have a problem with; you can always go to the boss's boss later. In any of these cases the advice is the same: do not rest your case on your word against the rater's.

If you are going to pit your opinion against the rater's, you will not have much of a chance of effecting any change. The only thing you might accomplish is to register your disagreement, which may be a meaningless gesture. What you need to challenge in an evaluation is evidence. You will need proof that what you say is really true and that somehow the rater did not know about it (and here it is often better not to blame anyone and just to call it an oversight so that the rater will be less defensive). To have this evidence may mean that you would have to have been collecting information before you knew you would be getting a substandard evaluation. People are told to drive defensively; maybe they need to work defensively too. It would certainly be much easier to collect supportive information before, rather than after, the fact. The information could include keeping copies of previous evaluations, letters from patients or clients complimenting your performance, or even a chronological, anecdotal record of your daily or weekly work. Supporting documents are more important for new employees, but even senior employees occasionally need them. Do not, however, rely on coworkers' testimony for support. The rater or reviewer of your case may not give them much credence unless they have very specific knowledge or have witnessed incidents that strongly support your case, and it takes a brave person to stand up to the boss with you, especially when there is little or no gain and perhaps significant risk for him or her.

Once you have your evidence, the final outcome may rest on your presentation. Here are some important suggestions:

- Remain calm and unemotional.
- Practice your statement.
- Present information in a logical order.
- Avoid accusations against the rater; try not to make him or her more defensive than he or she already is.
- Follow the conflict management guidelines presented in Chapter 3.
- Remain calm and unemotional.

Obviously remaining calm and unemotional is important because it was mentioned twice. The more rational and businesslike you appear, the more credibility you will have. An angry, emotional outburst filled with accusations is a good way to have yourself and your contentions discounted. State your case in positive, objective, nonthreatening terms, answer any questions in the same manner, get a date and time by which they will reply (in writing), and leave. Give the person or persons time to think, and, even if the rating is not changed, leave them thinking no less of you for having stated your case.

Summary

The evaluation process should not be the passive activity it has become in the minds of many managees. You must watch out for yourself and your good name as a health-care professional and as a professional employee. Remember that a performance evaluation involves one human being rating another, and this process is subject to all those failings that are human, along with some that may be intentional. Be in a position to defend your work, even if this means keeping track of your own performance (like keeping track of your work with each patient, client, or case, or at least trying to make sure you can identify and distinguish your work from that of others). If you do have to stand up for yourself, do so, but with the knowledge that there are risks even if you are correct. You will be the only person who can weigh these risks against possible benefits. Finally, if you do challenge an evaluation, make sure you follow company policy and make your claim in a professional, businesslike manner.

REFERENCES

1. Strauss, G, and Sayles, LR: Behavioral Strategies for Managers. Prentice-Hall, Englewood Cliffs, NJ, 1980, p 272.
2. Strauss and Sayles, p 272.

3. Strauss and Sayles, p 272.
4. Lowenburg, G, and Conrad, K: Current Perspectives in Industrial/Organizational Psychology. Allyn and Bacon, Needham Heights, Mass., 1998, p 181.
5. Daft, RL: Management, ed 5. Dryden, Fort Worth, 2000, p 414.
6. Lowenburg, and Conrad, p 181.
7. Strauss, and Sayles, p 273.
8. Strauss and Sayles, p 273.
9. Strauss and Sayles, p 273.
10. Lowenburg, and Conrad, p 166.
11. Vecchio, R: Organizational Behavior, ed 3. Dryden, Fort Worth, 1995, pp 87–91.
12. Lowenburg, and Conrad, p 182.

8 • Management Decisions: Understanding and Coping with Them

Objectives

On completion of this chapter, the reader will be able to:

☐ List and explain the decision-making process.

☐ Describe a managerial decision-making model.

☐ Identify the manager's and managee's roles in decision making.

☐ Be able to identify and describe decision coping strategies.

☐ Contrast the managee's decision-making role under classical and behavioral managers.

☐ Analyze and classify types of managerial decisions.

☐ List possible responses to adverse decisions.

As a managee, you can be involved in the organization's decision making in two general ways. First, you may be involved in the decision-making process itself. Second, some decisions will affect you. Being able to identify the type of decision may help you to better cope with it.

The Decision-making Process

Good managers will have a system for making decisions. Sometimes the system will be readily apparent. Other times the manager knows the system so well that it may appear that he or she is not using one at all. You, as a managee, may be involved at different levels depending on the decision and the manager's style. Here, we will identify the common areas where managees are involved and the level of involvement.

A DECISION-MAKING MODEL AND THE MANAGEE'S ROLE

The following is a typical decision-making model. The stages a managee may be involved with are marked by an asterisk:

1. * Identify that there is a problem.
2. Define the problem.
3. * List alternatives.
4. Evaluate alternatives.
5. Select an alternative.
6. * Implement the selection.
7. * Evaluate the results of the decision.

This decision-making model and its typical implementation by classical and behavioral managers is summarized in Table 8–1.

Problems must be identified before they can be solved.[1–4] It is in everyone's best interest that the health-care system work as well as possible—especially because patient care is the first priority. Therefore, everyone should help in identifying problems so that they may be corrected or changed as soon as possible. These problems include difficulties with equipment, supplies, and the work environment, as well as with people. At this point the managee's responsibility should be to identify and report problems. The manager's responsibility is to accept the reported problem, in a way that will *encourage*, not *discourage*, the person from reporting future problems, and to act on the problem immediately. Once a problem is identified, it must be clarified and defined.

Defining the problem is usually the manager's domain because he or she tries to ensure that the ensuing decision treats the problem and not just its symptom. Defining the problem involves investi-gating and clarifying it.[5,6] The problem must be stated completely, yet succinctly. Problem definition is a critical step if the problem is to be resolved. For example, a manager may discover a "problem" with tardiness and absenteeism. In fact, these are not problems but symptoms of some other problem. People do not come in late or miss work for no reason or just to be late or absent. Instead, the actual problem may be work related (poor equipment, insufficient staff for the workload, poor supervisor, and so on) or the problem may be personal (family problems, time-management problems, substance abuse problems, and so on). The manager must determine the real problem before compiling alternatives to solve it.

When *listing alternatives*, groups will usually generate more options than will an individual.[7] A behavioral manager will include frontline workers in alternative-generating groups.[8] Classical managers generally do not.[9] When participating in group alternative generation, you may be reluctant to put forth ideas. You may feel your ideas are unworthy or that your suggestions will be ignored. It is vital, however, that you respond when asked for input if you wish to continue to have a chance to influence decisions that may affect you. Managers are only human. If they ask for input and receive none, they will eventually stop asking. Thus, even if you feel your feedback will have no impact on the decision, respond. If you don't, it may be your last chance. If you do, you have encouraged the manager to ask again.

TABLE 8–1 • A DECISION-MAKING MODEL AND ITS TYPICAL IMPLEMENTATION BY CLASSICAL AND BEHAVIORAL MANAGERS

Decision-making Process	Classical Manager	Behavioral Manager
Identify the problem.	Through strict control mechanisms.	Through some control; feedback from managees.
Define the problem.	Symptom or problem? If symptom, manager finds an underlying problem.	Symptom or problem? If symptom, manager, and sometimes managees, finds underlying problem.
List alternatives.	Manager develops options.	Group (manager and managees) develops options.
Evaluate alternatives.	Manager weighs pros and cons.	Totally behavioral manager: Group weighs pros and cons. Partially behavioral manager: Manager weighs pros and cons of group's alternatives.
Decide; select an alternative.	Manager decides.	Totally behavioral manager: Group decides. Partially behavioral manager: Manager decides.
Implement the selection.	Usually by direct order.	Group consensus and participation.
Evaluate the results of the decision.	Manager evaluates.	Manager and managees evaluate.

The jobs of *evaluating alternatives* and *selecting one alternative* are generally the manager's.[10–12] He or she will usually have to weigh factors that are unknown or unfamiliar to managees. Also, the manager is almost always the person who will be held accountable for the results of the decision.[13,14] There are some situations in which a group decision is made by the manager and the managees. Here, all should share in the credit if the decision works well, just as all should share the responsibility for a decision that does not accomplish the desired effect.

Implementing decisions often involves managees.[15] This is one reason some managers include them in the step where alternatives are generated. People tend to accept changes more readily when they are involved in the process.[16] (Note, however, that managee participation in this or any stage of decision making does not guarantee cooperation. In fact, as will be seen in the section "Change," in Chapter 10, some people will resist implementation for many reasons and, in many ways, despite management's best efforts to anticipate and ward off such resistance.)

Finally, managees should be involved in *evaluating the results of the decision.*[17] The answer to the question "Did the decision solve the problem?" should be answered by all those affected by the decision.[18] Here, you should respond for the same reasons given for listing alternatives. If the decision did not solve the problem, the process should return to step 1.[19]

Coping with Decisions

Occasions to participate in decision making will vary depending on the manager's style and the situation. Whether you participate in the decision process or not, you will have many opportunities to cope with the results of decisions. The basic strategies for coping with decisions are escape, amnesia, and anger (Table 8–2).

ESCAPE

Escape is simple, but drastic. The person flees the situation by quitting, transferring, or being absent or tardy. The last choice sends signals that there is a problem, but the manager may not notice the signal. Even if he or she does notice, the manager may not change the decision. In addition, people are late or absent for reasons other than being unhappy with a decision, so the gesture may be futile. Quitting and transferring obviate the need for any further action by the manager or the managee.

AMNESIA

Some people are capable of forgetting about decisions they do not like. This amnesia can be active or passive. It is active when the person thinks about the situation and consciously decides to forget it. The amnesia is passive when the person doesn't care about much in general. The person does not review the situation because he or she just is not concerned with having to think about it at all.

ANGER

Other people get angry or upset when a decision has been made that is not in their favor or that adversely affects them. Some become very angry, whereas others view the decision as a source of irritation. In either case, the reaction can adversely affect the person's job performance or personal life, or both. Anger may not be an effective coping strategy, but it is a common one. When the anger lingers, it is a destructive strategy, especially when little can be done to change the decision. About all

TABLE 8–2 • BASIC STRATEGIES FOR COPING WITH DECISIONS
THAT A MANAGEE DOES NOT LIKE

Coping Strategy	Definition
Escape	Avoiding a decision's impact by quitting, transferring, being absent, or arriving late
Amnesia	Forgetting
Active	Consciously suppressing something
Passive	Not thinking about something
Anger	Becoming upset, irritated, or even enraged over a decision

 Building Comprehension Exercise begins on following page

BUILDING COMPREHENSION EXERCISE 8–1

Decision Making

There are 10 people in your department. Each is currently working full-time (scheduled for 40 hours per week). Paychecks are issued every 2 weeks. Management reports are generated every two pay periods. Each management report shows that the department is working 16 hours of overtime. Upper management has declared that the salary expenses must decrease by 10 percent. Follow the steps in the decision-making model to resolve this situation.

1. Identify the problem.

_____

_____

2. Define the problem.

_____

_____

3. List alternatives.

_____

_____

_____

_____

_____

_____

4. Evaluate alternatives.

_____

_____

_____

_____

_____

_____

Exercise continues on following page ⬡ ⬡ ⬡

5. Select an alternative.

_____

_____

_____

End of exercise. Text continues on following page.

that is accomplished is that the person gets upset. The manager may rarely, if ever, know of these feelings, and even if he or she does know, there may be little that the manager can do to change the decision. The remainder of this chapter is especially for people who have been upset by a management decision.

Classifying Decisions

When a decision is not to some people's liking, it is not uncommon for them to become so upset that they cannot work as well as they had in the past. They may also try to fix blame on the manager, the organization, themselves, coworkers, or others. Often, they speculate on the reason that the decision was made. As often as not, the reason they end up creating and believing is wrong, and they never know the real reason. Instead of trying to read the manager's mind or deduce the decision maker's motives for making a particular decision,

it is often easier to classify the decision, accept it for what it is, and be done with it.

I have developed eight general classes of decisions to help you categorize decisions. Hopefully you will be able to classify decisions that adversely affect you and put them behind you. The eight general types are rational, economic, political, emotional, temporal, risk based, conflict based, and buck passing (Table 8–3).

RATIONAL

Rational decisions are the type that people are supposed to make. They are logical and objective.[20] They do not take into account personalities, prejudice, and emotions.[21] They can be difficult for you to identify because doing so may mean you have to admit that someone was more qualified for the job you wanted or that it makes sense to give you the most difficult patients because you are best able to handle them at the time, and so on. However, if you can stand back, remove yourself from

TABLE 8–3 • EIGHT GENERAL CLASSES OF DECISIONS

Decision Type	Definition
Rational	Logical and objective
Economic	Financial or money based; whatever costs the least (typically meaning for the short term)
Political	To satisfy personal, rather than organizational, objectives
Popular	Satisfies the majority of the group members
Personal	Promotes manager's personal or career needs
Superior's	Satisfies the needs of the manager's boss
Rewarding	Returns a favor
Punishing	Penalizes actions the manager does not like
Emotional	Based on feelings or sentiment
Angry	Decision made when manager is mad or enraged
Affective	Based on emotions or instinct, other than anger; subjective, rather than objective
Temporal	Time based
Short time	Decisions that must be made fast
Emergency	A crisis situation; disaster is imminent
Quick	Instant, but nonemergency; pressure for an immediate decision comes more often from impatience than from a real crisis
Long time	Long, or longer than normal, time-based decisions
Delayed	Procrastinated decisions, often because it seems to be of less importance than other issues
Barrier	Conditions added to the situation that must be met before a decision can be made; designed to impede, rather than assist, decision making
Nondecision	Not deciding as a means of saying no
Risk based	Chance of loss or gain of utmost importance
Low risk	Little chance of failure or loss; safe
High risk	Great chance of loss; blame may be affixed on people other than the manager who made the high-risk decision
Conflict based	Involving a large potential to increase or decrease confrontations or discord
Buck passing	Avoiding a decision by having someone else make it or by allowing someone else to make it

the situation, and be objective, you may be able to see that, *from the decision maker's point of view,* his or her choice was the logical one to make.

Decisions are not always *perfect* because managers are only human. However, given the information available, managers try to make the best decision possible. When you try to classify a decision as logical, be careful that you do not assume the manager knows everything. Do not think, "She should have given me that job. She should have known I wanted it," when you have never mentioned being interested in it. Managers are not mind readers. Put yourself in the manager's position, and realize that many decisions are difficult to make. When people realize that a decision was a rational one, it is usually much easier for them to accept.

ECONOMIC

Economic decisions are those based solely on money.[22,23] These decisions can also be easy to accept because they are at least objective. One alternative is less expensive at the time than the others. The decision may not be rational or popular, but anyone can add up the numbers and see which course of action costs the least. Although people may accept the numerical facts, it can be much more difficult to accept the implications. This is especially true if the economic decision is to eliminate your position or to reduce your pay; however, realizing that this was a cold, hard business decision may at least save you from losing your self-esteem. If you are the last one hired and the first fired because of budget restrictions, don't blame yourself; instead, do everything you can to chalk it up to bad luck and move on. This process starts with accepting the economics of these situations.

POLITICAL

Although most decisions take into account organization politics, here the *political classification* refers to those decisions based almost exclusively on this one factor.[24] Furthermore, I divide political decisions into one of five subcategories: popular, personal, superior's, rewarding, and punishing.

Decisions that are politically *popular* are those made to satisfy the majority of the department.[25] Other concerns—economics, logic, and so on—may be ignored to do what the people want.

Personal political decisions are those made to foster the personal or career needs of the manager.[26] The needs of the department or of the organization are secondary to advancing the desires of the manager. These desires can be for power, control, advancement, transfer, leaving to another facility, and others. Obviously, it is difficult to accept a decision that adversely impacts you so that the manager can receive some personal gain, but it happens. Knowing that the decision was based on this and not your abilities (or lack thereof) may offer some comfort.

A *superior's* politics can cause managers to make decisions they ordinarily would not.[27] This involves the same things as when a manager makes a decision for his or her own gain except that the boss's needs are substituted for the manager's own. The net effect on you may be the same, but, for what it is worth, you know it wasn't your manager's doing, and that relationship need not change.

Some decisions are made just to *reward* someone for political support on other issues.[28,29] If someone else receives the promotion you applied for, it may be because they aided someone that was in a position to give them something later on. At least you will know that it wasn't you or some perceived inability that caused you not to get what you wanted.

Political *punishment* is another possibility. A decision may go against you to punish you, a coworker, your manager, or your department.[30,31] You may be punished for holding views contrary to the manager's or the organization's. Or you may have brought forth an issue that embarrassed a superior even though you were right. Sometimes you are punished for being too good at your job. If you are very good, a superior may feel that you threaten him or her; instead of moving you a step closer to taking her job, she may leave you in the front ranks—or move you further away.

EMOTIONAL

Emotional decisions can be divided into those arising from anger or from affective responses.[32] Here, decision makers rely on feelings, rather than rational thought. Sentiment, rather than logic, is their guide.

Decisions made in *anger* are obvious to see when made in your presence and more difficult when they are not.[33] The decision maker may, or may not, be angry with you. Sometimes managers make decisions that negatively affect you when the managers are actually angry with themselves, their spouses, their boss, or some other situation. If the decision was made in anger at you and to unjustly punish you, you may be able to file a complaint, or grievance, with the decision maker's superior or through the human resource department. If the manager made a decision that adversely affected you while he or she was angry at something else, then it is usually best to wait until he or she is no longer mad and ask for reconsideration. Going over the manager's head in this situation, before talking to him or her, is probably unwise.

Decisions made in anger seem to be the most common of the emotional type. Other emotion-based decisions are in the *affective* category. This includes decisions made according to "instinct," "gut reaction," and other subjective situational reactions.[34] To counter these decisions, ask why the decision was made. "Because I said so" is not a sufficient answer. There should be a logical, concrete reason. Recognize, however, that there are times when a manager may be required to select one of two equal alternatives—the "six of one, half dozen of another" kind of decisions—but they are not all of this kind. Unfortunately, some of these "gut" decisions are made in hiring people. Even when you believe you were discriminated against, it is difficult to prove and time- and money-consuming to pursue. About the only solace you may receive is in knowing you were not held up to rational evaluation and found lacking.

TEMPORAL

Temporal, or time-based, decisions range from those made in a short amount of time to those that take a long time.[35] Both have subtypes. I categorize short-time decisions as "emergency" and "quick." Decisions taking a long time are the "delayed," "barrier," and the "nondecision."

In *emergency situations* there is high pressure to make fast decisions.[36] In these situations, a less-than-ideal choice should be forgiven.[37] If everyone could make good, rational decisions instantly, they would. The fact is that most decisions require information and some thought. In emergency situations there may not be time for one or both of these. Unless there are major ramifications, and I would say that most emergency decisions do not cause these, it is probably best to forgive and forget poor decisions made in these uncommon situations.

Decisions are often made on the spur of the moment in nonemergency conditions.[38] *Quick major decisions* can be poor ones if the decision maker does not have adequate time to research or think about the problem. Sometimes managers make quick decisions on their own; sometimes managees press the manager for a fast decision. The majority of the time this is unwise. Do not ask for, or worse yet, demand, a fast judgment because the result may be a fast decision against you or an angry, fast decision. Sometimes the man-

ager may just say no because there is an old management maxim that says, "Always say no because you can change it to yes later, but not vice versa." Do what you can to give the manager time to think and decide. If it seems like he or she is going to make a snap decision, you can volunteer not to need a decision for a couple of days, allowing the manager the time to, hopefully, come to your decision.

Delayed decisions seem to be drawn out forever. If the decision maker never mentions the subject to you and never seems to have a reason for not making the decision, he or she may be trying to delay the decision in the hope that you will forget about it.[39] If you think this may be happening, you can casually inquire about when to expect the decision to be made. Try to get a date or time from the manager. Try not to let him or her be vague. The frequency of your reminders must be based on your own judgment. Some managers might get annoyed at frequent inquiries and make an angry decision that might not be to your liking. However, some managers will give you the decision you want just to get rid of you.

Barrier decisions are those decisions that are delayed because the decision maker continually adds new conditions, or barriers, that must be met before a decision can even be attempted.[40] One common tactic is to tell a person that any request must be in writing. This may or may not involve a form of some kind. Another tactic is that the decision maker will not be able to make a decision until some other thing occurs—a report must come out, you must perform at a certain level, it must be your anniversary date, the new fiscal year must begin, and so on. Almost always this other condition is beyond the decision maker's control. Whatever the reason is, the effect is to place another obstacle in your path before a decision can be made. The decision maker's hope is that all of these impediments will wear you down and you will go away. Then no decision will be required, the decider will have effectively said no without having to speak the word (and they are no longer accountable or responsible for saying no), and the status quo is maintained.

The *nondecision* drags out so long that it never really gets made. Choosing not to decide is another form of saying no and maintaining the status quo without actually having to say the word "no."[41] Some managers may use a form of the word "no" when they say, "We are not able to make a decision regarding this at this time." When this is said, you may have to accept it as a "no" and proceed from there. If nothing is ever said again, then you may have learned something about your status in the organization—that it is not too high.

RISK BASED

Some managers base their decisions on the amount of *risk* involved.[42] Of these, there are two extremes. One will agree to make only low-risk decisions, that is, those with little chance of failure or in which failure would not be visible to superiors or people outside the department.[43] At the opposite extreme are those who are too willing to agree to high risks.[44] They are seemingly unconcerned with failure or the visibility of failure. However, if a situation gets out of control, they may point the blame at you or find themselves out of a job (sometimes taking you with them).

With managers who only agree to low-risk decisions, you must show how you have accounted for any risks or at least how you have brought the risks down to a reasonable level. With high-risk decision makers, you should make sure that someone has managed the risks. If the manager doesn't, you may have to, to cover yourself.

CONFLICT BASED

Decisions may also be made based on the *conflict* they cause or reduce.[45] Some decisions *minimize conflict* between managees.[46] Although doing the popular thing can often minimize conflict, this peace-keeping strategy is a form of political decision making, as mentioned earlier. In addition, sometimes minimal-conflict decisions have a personal side.[47] A decision may be made against a particular person simply because he or she is the least likely to complain about it, perhaps because he is just not the kind of person to complain or speak out, or because she is not in a position to speak out. Or one employee may be singled out because he or she is new or needs the job more than others or because he or she has not been performing well and does not want to upset the manager any more than necessary by making waves.

Some managers make decisions that they know will *cause* conflict because they may wish that a particular employee will quit as a result, which would thus eliminate the need for the manager to fire him or her.[48] Other managers believe that a certain level of chronic conflict between managees is beneficial because it will "keep them sharp" or "on their toes." If the level of conflict is not there naturally, these managers will introduce conflict-generating decisions.[49] It is unlikely that this strategy actually motivates employees over the long term. However, it is safe to assume that such ongoing conflict will certainly keep managees from banding together in a potentially powerful informal organization.

BUCK PASSING

The final category is the decision to let someone else make the decision. *Passing the buck* means to send the decision to someone else, thereby avoiding it and the responsibility for it.[50] There are situations in which the decision must be made at another level. There are also situations in which the manager is hoping that by passing the decision along, he or she will avoid having to deal with it and the managee will lack the perseverance to address the matter further. It will be dropped, and the status quo—which the manager wanted all along—will be maintained. If the matter is important enough to you, do not allow this tactic to work. Pursue the decision. Pursue it calmly and rationally, but pursue it until you have a definite answer.

Summary

As a managee, decisions that managers make will affect you—sometimes positively, sometimes not. When a decision is made that you do not like, you may try to get the decision changed. Often this is impractical, unlikely, or unwise. The classes of decisions and possible responses have been described. For those times when your response is anger, it may be helpful to classify the decision, accept it for what it is, and move on. To become upset, bitter, or to dwell on an unfavorable decision frequently changes nothing and takes a toll only on you. It is usually better to leave it behind you and get on with your life, work, and career.

REFERENCES

1. Griffin, RW: Management, ed 6. Houghton Mifflin, Boston, 1999, p 206.
2. Bateman, TS, and Zeithaml, CP: Management: Function and Strategy, ed 2. Irwin, Homewood, Ill., 1993, p 89.
3. Dilworth, J: Operations Management, ed 3. Dryden, Fort Worth, 2000, p 64.
4. Higgins, JM: The Management Challenge. Macmillan, New York, 1991, p 76.
5. Griffin, p 206.
6. Stevenson, W: Production Operations Management, ed 6. Irwin/McGraw-Hill, Boston, 1999, p 64.
7. Dilworth, p 65.
8. Vecchio, R: Organizational Behavior, ed 3. Dryden, Fort Worth, 1995, pp 402–05.
9. Daft, RL: Management, ed 5. Dryden, Fort Worth, 2000, pp 272–73.
10. Bateman, and Zeithaml, p 91.
11. Stoner, JAF, and Freeman, RE: Management, ed 5. Prentice-Hall, Englewood Cliffs, NJ, 1992, p 56.
12. Daft, pp 280–81.
13. Griffin, p 210.
14. Daft, p 268.

15. Dilworth, p 63.
16. Nelson, D, and Quick, J: Organizational Behavior. West, St. Paul, 1994, pp 306–07.
17. Griffin, p 211.
18. Bateman, and Zeithaml, p 93.
19. Stevenson, p 64.
20. Griffin, p 206.
21. Nelson, and Quick, p 297.
22. Mosley, DC, et al: Supervisory Management—The Art of Empowering and Developing People, ed 5. Southwestern Publishing, Cincinnati, 2001, p 69.
23. Higgins, p 88.
24. Griffin, p 213.
25. Mosley, et al, p 77.
26. Griffin, p 410.
27. Aldag, RJ, and Stearns, TM: Management, ed 2. Southwestern Publishing, Cincinnati, 1991, p 340.
28. Griffin, p 410.
29. Chapman, EN: Supervisor's Survival Kit, ed 6. Macmillan, New York, 1993, p 214.
30. Griffin, p 44.
31. Bateman, and Zeithaml, p 414.
32. Mosley, et al, p 71.
33. Bateman, and Zeithaml, p 102.
34. Griffin, p 214.
35. Daughtrey, AS, and Ricks, BR: Contemporary Supervision—Managing People and Technology, ed. 2. McGraw-Hill, New York, 1994, p 98.
36. Griffin, p 203.
37. Daughtrey, and Ricks, p 100.
38. Rue, LW, and Byars, LL: Supervision, ed 4. Irwin, Homewood, Ill., 1993, p 39.
39. Bateman, and Zeithaml, p 102.
40. Mosley, et al, p 71.
41. Chapman, p 190.
42. Bateman, and Zeithaml, p 88.
43. Mosley, et al, p 69.
44. Griffin, p 205.
45. Bateman, and Zeithaml, p 88.
46. Mosley, et al, p 72.
47. Bateman, and Zeithaml, p 96.
48. Rue, and Byars, p 37.
49. Aldag, and Stearns, p 556.
50. Daughtrey, and Ricks, p 100.

9 • Understanding Motivation

Objectives

On completion of this chapter, the reader will be able to:

☐ Describe and differentiate the various motivational theorists.
☐ Describe the application of the major motivational theories to the health professions.
☐ Identify the various types of motivational techniques.
☐ Describe management's view of motivation.
☐ Describe advantages to managees for participating in their own motivational management.
☐ Describe methods for managees to take a more active role in their motivational management.
☐ Enable the reader to identify motivational methods that are being used by a manager.

There are three reasons why managees should know the motivational theories managers are taught to use:

1. The theories were developed in an attempt to understand managees. Each theorist was trying to understand what made people produce. Understanding motivational theories may help you to understand what does and does not motivate you, and why.

2. If you know the various motivational theories, you can identify which one your manager is using. This knowledge allows you to identify the assumptions the manager is making and enables you to coordinate your motivationally related request with the manager's theory. Knowing the theory or theories being used by your manager may also help you to identify managers you wish to work for and

may identify areas of conflict if your motivational style does not match your manager's.

3. If these theories are going to be employed in an attempt to alter your behavior (and that is their real purpose), you should know what their tactics are.

Motivational Theorists

For purposes of study and identification, the major theorists have been divided into three categories. The classicalists are associated with the classical school of management thought. They were some of the first people to formulate an organized theory of motivation. The behavioralists are allied with the behavioral, or human relations, managers. Basically, they formed these theories as management's response to the failings and abuse of the classical theories. The contemporaneous theories are generally those that can be used along with any other theory. Many of these have been developed only recently.

THE CLASSICALISTS

The classicalists' theories began to be formulated in the late 1800s and early 1900s. Their names and theories are summarized in Table 9–1. There are three major early classical writers. Fayol, Weber, and Taylor. Henri Fayol, working in France, was actually an organizational theorist. His organizational theories, however, contained motivation-related concepts. He also classified management functions as planning, coordinating, controlling, organizing, and directing—differentiations that are still used today. He also described some basic guidelines for managers. Max Weber (pronounced Váy-ber) was a German whose main area was also organization theory. Like Fayol, his writings had motivational components. The third early theorist was an American, Frederick Taylor, generally considered to be the originator of classical, and even modern, management.

Henri Fayol

In addition to dividing management functions into separate categories, Fayol detailed some basic principles for managers. Some, from the chapter on management (see Chap. 5), will be familiar. Most, if not all, are still valid today, although they are not used by all managers. Those concerning motivation include:

- Division of labor
- Unity of command
- Subordination of interests
- Remuneration
- Equity[1,2]

As will be seen, the effect of each of these varies. Some affect motivation negatively, others positively.

Actually, *division of labor*, or specialization, predates Fayol by many years. In the 1700s Adam

TABLE 9–1 • THE CLASSICALISTS' THEORIES (FORMULATED IN THE LATE 1800s AND EARLY 1900s)

Henri Fayol	From France, was actually writing about organization theory. He is known for recording many of the principles of management. His efforts to increase the efficiency and working of organizations directly affected motivation.
Max Weber	From Germany, he was mainly an organization theorist like Fayol. Created the bureaucracy. Many of his concepts (hire and promote people based on their qualifications, and so on) provide motivation to many. His separation principle has led to a lessening of the value that is placed on managees by managers.
Fredrick Taylor	The "Father of Scientific (classical) Management." Although Fayol and Weber predate him, he is considered the first management theorist, as opposed to an organizational theorist. Basic motivator was money, especially paid by a piece rate. Taylor specialized in time studies to increase the rate at which people worked, thereby increasing their pay.
Henry Gantt	Continued the work of Taylor. Motivated by paying a piece rate but modified the concept. His system paid a wage for a standard day's work and a bonus for exceeding the standard. A bonus wage was paid to the managee and the manager. He felt this development would encourage managers to teach their managees how to work faster.
Lilian and Frank Gilbreth	Continued the work of Taylor. Motivated by money. Used time-motion studies to eliminate wasted movements, thus increasing speed. Applied their management ideas to their family of 12 children. Featured in the movie *Cheaper by the Dozen*.

Smith extolled the virtues of this principle in *The Wealth of Nations,* in which he described the workings in a pin factory. Advocates of division of labor point out, correctly, that it increases efficiency and productivity. It also makes people experts in their areas. However, if the job is divided into tasks that are highly repetitive and essentially identical, specialization can lead to boredom. Therefore, managers have developed the concepts of job enlargement, job enrichment, and job rotation in an attempt to counteract some of the motivationally negative effects of the division of labor. *Job enlargement* means adding tasks at the same level of difficulty or involvement. *Job enrichment* means adding difficulty or involvement (such as self-checking) to the same job. *Job rotation* involves people trading positions for variety. Fayol recommended division of labor for managers too.

The division-of-labor principle is widely applied in health care, as evidenced in the number of health-care specialties and subspecialties. Division of labor is also vital in the health-care industry because of the wide diversity of knowledge required in the various health fields. To apply job enlargement to the health fields, specialists in one field would have to learn another. For years this practice was common in radiology. Technologists learned radiography and nuclear medicine or radiography and radiation therapy. Applying job enrichment would mean that a health specialist would increase his or her depth of knowledge within the same field. Often this involves training health-care professionals to check their own work or monitor their own quality. Job enrichment could also involve additional training within one health specialty. Job rotation would involve rotating employees among different assignments within one health specialty.

Fayol's principle of *unity of command* states that a person should have only one boss. Conflicting orders, differing standards and expectations, and confusion—all rather unmotivating—can result when you have more than one manager. Unfortunately, many health professions partially violate the unity-of-command principle because they have an administrative department head to handle management-related tasks and a physician to handle medical tasks. Close coordination is required between these two positions so that they do not work against each other.

The *subordination-of-interests principle* states that the organization's goals are more important than those of any individual. The company should be put first. Having your goals aligned with the organization's can help motivate you. When your goals are not similar to the company's, there is no motivational effect. Subordination of interests is the rule among health-care professionals because all are taught that the patient comes first.

Fayol professed *fair remuneration* for everyone in the company. Of course, money and benefits are important to all employees. They motivate people to work in the first place. Opportunities to increase reimbursement also motivate some people (others seek different rewards). Some of the theorists described later in this chapter feel that remuneration can motivate only to a certain point. However, most agree with Fayol that when pay is *not* adequate or *not* fairly distributed among the different levels of employees, motivation is actually reduced. When remuneration is not fairly distributed, employees may feel that working hard, or even adequately, is futile because the rewards do not coincide with their efforts.

Fayol's *equity principle* states that managers should be just and kind toward managees. Fair and friendly treatment is not only human decency but is also felt to be motivational. These and Fayol's other principles were intended to be a guide for managers to use while also pursuing efficiency, order, and stability. In the hands of some, the work environment embodies these principles, but in others, it becomes rigid and inflexible.

Max Weber

Max Weber worked in Germany in the late 1800s and early 1900s and wrote only in German. His work was not translated into English until about 1940. Because of this he was late in being credited with having devised some classical precepts. Weber created what he thought was an ideal form of organization. He devised the bureaucracy. Although he did foresee some problems with it, he never envisioned the modern interpretation of a bureaucracy as something slow, inefficient, and difficult to work with.

Weber's system has had a profound effect on the working environment and motivation. The aspects having the greatest effect include his principles of:

- Hierarchical structure
- Division of labor
- Rules and regulations
- Technical competence
- Separation[3]

Although, like Fayol, Weber was actually an organizational theorist, he believed that organizations are composed of people; therefore, they affect all employees.

Weber stressed the *hierarchical structure* (pyramid-shaped chain of command) for organizations to facilitate the control of employees. Although all organizations have a chain of command, Weber favored one with a narrow span of control; thus there were many managers, each controlling only a few managees. This made close supervision possible. In practice, uniformity of production did increase, but flexibility often decreased.

Hierarchical structures have two opposite effects on motivation. The opportunity to "climb" the organization's "ladder" toward greater power and money increased motivation for some. For those who knew they would not be moving up (that they would stay where they were or move down the ladder), no motivation was provided. Also, it was not motivational when the close supervision of the small work groups became an inflexible, rigid system, or when individual workers who could function independently were subject to close scrutiny.

Weber, like others, had a *division-of-labor principle,* but he believed that tasks must be broken down into the smallest divisions possible. He felt this would increase efficiency and reduce training times for new workers. Both are generally true; however, repeating the same limited number of tasks does not provide much motivation.

Weber's system relied on rules to ensure uniformity, conformity, and stability. The people might come and go, but the rules would be there to ensure continuity. This approach does not provide much motivation for those who are innovators or have their own way of doing things.

Weber believed in selecting employees based not on friendship or nepotism but on *technical competence.* Weber believed that a job should be described; then the type of education, abilities, and experience needed by a person to fill this position should be listed. As candidates presented themselves, one only needed to match the requirements to the personal facts and to seek the best match. The process was meant to be objective and unbiased. By matching the person to the task, Weber believed, employees would be motivated and would perform efficiently. Some motivational effect was also to be gained from applicants' knowing that the position would be awarded based on *what* they knew, not *who* they knew. Weber's ideas directly led to job analysis, job descriptions, and job specifications.

Possibly the principle with the greatest effect but the least often explained is that of *separation.* Weber said that the position in the organization that someone held and the person holding it are separate. This idea is related to that of technical competence. The job description describes the work, and the job specification defines the type of person who can do the work. The completion of the work is not dependent on any *one* person. Anybody with the specifications will be able to do an adequate job as outlined in the description.

The motivational effect here is so subtle that many, if not most, people are unaware of it—at least consciously. People may also be unaware of the subtle motivational influence because the principle is applied to different degrees in different organizations. Essentially, it says that you, as a person, do not matter to the functioning of the organization. Any other person having credentials like yours (that is, who meets the job specification) will be able to do the work. This can lead people to feel that they are not important or wanted by the organization. Many organizations that claim to care about individual employees in fact feel that people are easily replaceable. Thus, they are willing to go only so far to keep people. This principle also leads some managers to the attitude of "if you don't like your job, quit" because all the manager needs to do is to find another person who meets your position's job specification. Not all organizations function this way. It is important to know which kind of organization is which.

In summary, Weber was a rationalist. He believed in moving organizations to a logically efficient method of operation. Although he did not write about motivation, his organization theories affected beliefs about motivation. The fact that his principles are adhered to today makes them relevant for the purposes here.

Fredrick Taylor

Although many of Fayol's and Weber's ideas affected management and motivation, their primary focus was organization theory. Fredrick Taylor is commonly recognized as the first management theorist, per se. He believed that managers should take a scientific approach to studying work, and he called his collective theories *scientific management.* He had four main principles, three of which relate to motivation:

1. Find the critical elements of each task.
2. Offer monetary incentives.
3. Use functional foremanship.[4]

Finding the critical elements of each task through time studies was Taylor's way of determining the one best way to do each job. Through careful observation he would find the most efficient way of working. His concern was to increase productivity

 Building Comprehension Exercise begins on following page

BUILDING COMPREHENSION EXERCISE 9–1

Recognizing Principles of Management

Cite an example from your clinical site or your workplace that either supports (or illustrates) or contradicts (or refutes) each of these principles of management.

Division of Labor Principle _The coordinators at my fw site specialized in M.D_

Unity of Command Principle _At the MDA camp there was one camp director that was in charge of the camp itself_

Subordination of Interests Principle _At the MDA camp the goal was to give the kids the best week and to do what they want_

Equity Principle _My fw supervisors always treated me c̄ respect and helped c̄ anything I needed._

Hierarchical Structure Principle _My current job has one store supervisor c̄ multiple managers below him and supervisors below them_

Rules Principle _At the camp we had to follow rules to get the children to the activities, meals, showers and bed in_

a timely manner

Technical Competence Principle _My interview c̄ the MDA camp aligned me c̄ my camper because of common interests I also had specific requirements I had to meet_

Separation Principle _My current job is always replacing or training people to do other tasks so that if someone leaves they have replacements._

End of exercise. Text continues on following page.

and wages, and improve working conditions. His ways would benefit not only the company but also the workers. Some of his methods were designed to increase the speed of the workers, but others to reduce fatigue, stress, or injuries.[5]

The increased remuneration and reduction of fatigue and injuries did increase motivation, especially in the early, pay-oriented days of the industrial era. On the other hand, once the one best way for each task was discovered, all workers were expected to use it. Reducing flexibility was demotivating to some. Of even greater consequence was the fear Taylor's methods produced.

Although his work had positive benefits, many workers were afraid that the increased demand for output would result in managees working harder and managers and owners getting richer. Unfortunately, they were right. Many managers corrupted Taylor's methods. They used them to increase production, but they did not use the pay incentives. Taylor was actually called before Congress, where he explained that his methods would work only if workers and owners shared in the benefits, instead of just the owners.

The fear created by the abuses of unscrupulous managers and owners is still present today. Many work environments have unwritten standards of performance set by the informal organization. Exceeding these standards is greatly discouraged for fear that management will find out just how fast a job can really be done and make a new, higher standard for everyone. People that exceed the informal rate are called *rate busters,* and they are generally informed quickly about what the prevailing rate is. Although this situation does not motivate people to do their best, and the resulting inefficiency can eventually hurt everyone, one can hardly blame the workers, given the history of labor relations (see Chap. 6).

Not only did Taylor devise methods to increase productivity, but he advocated *offering monetary incentives* to work harder. Taylor devised a piece-rate system to motivate people, in which workers are paid a certain amount for each item they make or each task they complete. The faster one worked, the more one made. This practice did work in some cases. However, as mentioned before, some managers did not fully employ the system, to their gain and the workers' loss.[6]

Using functional foremanship meant that different managers were responsible for different phases of production. Workers fell under control of the manager responsible for the function—for example, planning or evaluating the work. This tended to decrease motivation because workers were relegated to just performing the work. The other tasks, like inspecting the work, were the concerns of managers.

Although some of Taylor's ideas came into widespread use, especially when combined with mass-production techniques, his system was not highly popular in America. His ideas as a whole did find acceptance in some European countries, however.[7]

Henry Gantt

Taylor and Gantt worked together employing Taylor's methods. Eventually Gantt felt that Taylor's ideas needed fine-tuning. Instead of a strict piece-rate system, Gantt devised a quota system with a bonus for exceeding it. If a worker did not make the quota, he or she was given a flat rate for the day. If the quota was exceeded, he or she received a bonus. The immediate superior would also receive a bonus so he or she would have an incentive to teach and motivate the workers to exceed the set minimum. Gantt, like Taylor, felt that efficiency or production was the prime concern for managers. But Gantt was also concerned with the worker's job satisfaction. His pay system was devised to increase satisfaction, which he felt would then motivate the workers to increase production.[8,9]

Lilian and Frank Gilbreth

The Gilbreths were a husband and wife team who were early believers in Taylor's theories. The Gilbreths' contribution was to add motion study to Taylor's time studies. Rather than devise ways that employees could work faster, the Gilbreths increased production by eliminating unnecessary motions. This also reduced fatigue. Possibly the biggest contribution to motivation by the Gilbreths was their idea of job rotation. They felt variety would decrease boredom and increase morale and satisfaction.[10,11]

The classical theories are still followed by managers, and the classicalists made important contributions to some of the foundations of management and motivation. On the other hand, they were also criticized on a number of points. For one, most of their experiences were from manufacturing situations. Second, some of the theorists made assumptions based on their opinions, not on scientific research. For example, they felt that workers should not, and did not, bring their personal lives, worries, and problems to work. This is not true for most people. They also assumed that people were motivated almost exclusively by money. Third, their rational system approach stressed formality and ignored the informal organization. Fourth, classical systems are not usually fast to respond to change; they are more suited to conditions that are fairly constant. Finally, classical theories give the impression that people are simply tiny cogs in a large machine—they do their jobs, are easily replaceable, and perform obediently.

Strict adherence to only classical motivation methods is not advisable for health-care situations. It must be remembered that all of the classicalists discussed here worked near the end of the 1800s and beginning of the 1900s. Those times and certainly the expectations of workers were vastly different from the present. Today, health workers are under pressure to work more efficiently in changing conditions, make independent decisions, and simultaneously deliver quality care. The classicalist theories do, however, have contributions to make to modern health-care management and motivation. Health-care managers could do their patients or clients, managees, and organizations a service if they applied some time-motion studies toward identifying and eliminating unnecessary movements. What is really needed is a blend of classical and behavioral theories.

THE BEHAVIORALISTS

The classical methods certainly have a place but also limitations and areas they do not address. Eventually, as workers and workplaces changed, there were two responses to these limitations and unaddressed areas. As mentioned in Chapter 5, one response by the workers was to form unions. Managers also noticed the deficiencies, and, because motivation theories try to accurately reflect reality, new theories and an entire new school of management thought were created.

Elton Mayo

Chapter 5 also detailed the beginnings of behavioral management, which began with the interpretations of the Hawthorne studies by Elton Mayo.[12] The general conclusion Mayo came to was that there is more to work than just the work. People work to satisfy a number of needs, not just the need for money. Thus motivation can be achieved through means other than wages and benefits, and satisfaction is affected by more than just remuneration.

As Mayo's conclusions became known, others contributed their ideas, and the behavioral school of management thought was born (Table 9–2).

Mary Parker Follett

One of Mary Parker Follett's[13] areas of study was conflict. Her major contribution to the resolution of conflicts, including those regarding motivation, was the idea of integration. According to Follett, the only satisfactory method for solving problems was to have both the manager and the managee work together. They were to work not as adversaries but as partners trying to find a solution to a shared problem. Therefore, managers should not only work with managees, they should also enlist their aid in problem solving and solicit their ideas.[14]

Douglas McGregor

McGregor[15] may not have been good at naming his theories, but he did summarize both the classical and behavioral systems and endorsed behavioralism. McGregor chose to call his outline of

TABLE 9–2 • MAJOR BEHAVIORAL THEORISTS

Elton Mayo	Australian professor from Harvard University. Assembled a team to interpret the Hawthorne studies and concluded that there is more to work than money and that people work for social purposes also. This marked the beginning of the behavioral school of management.
Mary Parker Follett	Studied conflict and concluded that the best way to resolve conflict was with the manager and managee working together.
Douglas McGregor	Differentiated classical and behavioral management, calling them "Theory X" and "Theory Y." Favored Theory Y (behavioral management).
Chris Argyris	Continued the work begun by the Hawthorne experiments; believed that the strict controls of classical management created workers who were passive and dependent so that rather than management's *responding* to "lazy" workers, strict management *created* "lazy" workers.
Abraham Maslow	Created the Hierarchy of Needs to explain motivation and how different things motivate some people but not others.
Fredrick Herzberg	Differentiated between hygiene factor (dissatisfiers) and motivators (satisfiers). Believed that adequate hygiene factors would eliminate dissatisfaction; adequate motivators would lead to satisfaction.

TABLE 9–3 • MCGREGOR'S THEORY X AND THEORY Y STYLES OF MANAGEMENT

Theory X, Classical	Theory Y, Behavioral
Work is disliked.	It is possible for workers to enjoy work.
Workers do not want responsibility.	Workers can play an important part in decision making.
Money is the prime motivator.	Workers will accept responsibility.
Workers are watched closely.	
Rules and control are emphasized.	

classical ideas "Theory X," and he called behavioral concepts "Theory Y." McGregor's theories are outlined in Table 9–3. McGregor believed that people could be motivated by things other than money.[16] He felt that involvement with the organization, through participation in decision making, would not only motivate workers but would benefit the organization. He felt that most workers could make a contribution, and that most wanted to contribute.[17]

Chris Argyris

Chris Argyris[18] questioned some of the basic tenets of classical motivation and job satisfaction theories and amplified the Hawthorne experiments. He said that, because classical managers controlled workers so closely, the workers became incapable of acting independently. Because most of the time workers were not allowed to think for themselves, they became uninterested in doing so during the rare occasions when they could have or when it would have been advantageous for the company for them to have. Argyris further said that lack of involvement and lack of opportunity for independent thought and action frustrated workers. This caused them to quit or to work against the organization's goals. Argyris felt that as people matured, they desired independence, more variety in their activities, and more control over their own actions. To give them these things would motivate them. To treat them as immature and ignore these factors would demotivate them.[19]

Abraham Maslow

Maslow's[20] Hierarchy of Needs is discussed in Chapter 1 and is summarized in Table 9–4. In Chapter 1, this hierarchy was mentioned as a way of explaining why people work. The concepts can also be used to motivate people. According to Maslow, any need that is unfulfilled can be used as a motivator.[21] One must only find the things that would satisfy a particular person's need. On the other hand, once a need is fulfilled, it can no longer be used to motivate.[22] For example, if a person has his or her physiologic, safety, and belonging needs met, he or she can be motivated if offered opportunities to fulfill status and self-esteem needs. It would be better to offer this person recognition or a new title rather than something from the lower three needs. Once the self-esteem and status needs are met, it would be less effective to try to motivate someone through personal awards or a mention in the hospital employee newsletter. According to Maslow, the self-actualizing need should be appealed to next. Offering new challenges or tuition reimbursement or work time for learning might be some ways to appeal to self-actualization.[23]

TABLE 9–4 • SUMMARY OF MASLOW'S HIERARCHY OF NEEDS

Need	Summary
Self-actualization	Need to achieve the most one can possibly achieve
Status and Self-esteem	Need for prestige, self-confidence, self-respect, pride in oneself
Belonging	Need to socialize (be with friends, other people) and the need for a mate
Safety	Need to feel safe and secure from harm
Physiologic	Need for food, shelter, clothing, and water

BUILDING COMPREHENSION EXERCISE 9–2

Using Maslow's Hierarchy

You can use Maslow's hierarchy by first determining your location on the hierarchy. Next, you can look toward fulfilling unmet needs. Realize, though, that not all needs can be met through work. If your need for status is unfulfilled and cannot be filled at work, look to other activities.

Where are you on Maslow's Hierarchy? Fill in or highlight each bar according to how well satisfied you are at each level.

Self-actualization Needs	10%	20%	30%	40%	50%	60%	70%	80%	90%	100%
Status and Self-esteem Needs	10%	20%	30%	40%	50%	60%	70%	80%	90%	100%
Belonging Needs	10%	20%	30%	40%	50%	60%	70%	80%	90%	100%
Safety Needs	10%	20%	30%	40%	50%	60%	70%	80%	90%	100%
Physiologic Needs	10%	20%	30%	40%	50%	60%	70%	80%	90%	100%

Which level of Maslow's needs will motivate you? _____

_____

How can these needs be used to motivate you? _____

_____

_____

Exercise continues on following page 🎲 🎲 🎲

Which of Maslow's needs can be satisfied for you through your chosen health profession and how? How might you meet these needs outside of your profession (see also Table 9–4).

	Needs met through profession	*How needs might be met outside of your profession*
Self-actualization Needs		
Status and Self-esteem Needs		
Belonging Needs		
Safety Needs		
Physiologic Needs		

End of exercise. Text continues on following page.

Fredrick Herzberg

Herzberg[24] divides work factors into two groups. He calls one group the "hygiene factors" and the other "motivators." According to Herzberg, *hygiene factors* do not motivate people when they are present, but if they are absent, they cause dissatisfaction. They are things like reimbursement (salary and benefits), a good supervisor, working conditions, work rules, and seniority benefits. Herzberg says that having a nice manager will not motivate you. On the other hand, if he or she treats you poorly, you will be unhappy—and not motivated. To be motivated, one of Herzberg's *motivators* must be used, and he recommended that they be used in conjunction with job enrichment.[25] Herzberg's motivators include achievement, recognition, responsibility, advancement, growth, and the work itself.[26] According to Herzberg's theory, when these are offered as rewards, people will motivate themselves to achieve them. Once they are earned, the person feels genuine satisfaction. Herzberg goes on to say that every job should be a learning experience and contain feedback for the person, and the individual should have the responsibility for self-checking the work (rather than having inspectors).[27]

In general, the behavioralists shed light on the importance of nonmonetary motivators. They investigated the social and psychological aspects of work. The value of the managees' input and their need to feel that they are more than just a piece of machinery was stressed. The behavioralists did not, however, answer all the questions regarding motivation and humans at work. Whenever people's psyches are involved, the task is complex. For one, money affects people differently, especially when salaries are low. The need for money can also vary with a person's lifestyle. When first beginning a career, money may be the main reason for working. People generally start out with little after leaving home. Because many do not immediately marry, their careers and financial conditions may improve and material needs may be met, to the point that money is less important. People in this situation may be better motivated by interesting work. If such a person should later marry and begin a family, then money may increase in importance to the point that it can once again be used to motivate.

Another reason that behavioral management's motivational techniques were not seen as perfect was that some managers' attempts at using behavioral techniques were so transparent that they were seen as being manipulative, and their attempts failed. Finally, the proof that a happier worker, or one treated according to behavioral principles, was a more productive worker has been less than over-whelming. It has not been proved beyond a doubt that treating workers nicely increases productivity. On the other hand, treating workers nicely has not decreased productivity either. So there is no reason for managers not to treat people as managees, rather than subordinates.[28]

A number of behavioral theories can and should be used in the health professions. One major theoretical area is a subject found in almost every book on health care—the health-care team. Yet how often are behavioral, group management, and team-building principles used? Sometimes they are used within departments, but they are not often used with members of different health professions. And almost no effort is expended toward team building with physicians, nurses, and other health professionals.

Another area of application could be the use of the managees' knowledge and experience in problem solving. In every health profession a certain amount of independent thought and judgment is required. Occupational therapists, physical therapists, and assistants in these fields may have to decide how far, or not, to push a client on a particular day. A radiographer has to decide if a patient can be placed upright or must remain recumbent. Every health-care worker may be faced with the decision to call for additional assistance or not.

Health professionals are trained to be self-reliant within the framework of their professions. Yet when it comes to reorganizing the department or planning or cutting costs, the workers may not be consulted. I contend that once people are trained to think, they continue to do so. I also contend that health workers are a little different from other workers. I believe they are in these jobs less for the money and more for the intrinsic satisfaction of helping others. Because of this, I believe that they are concerned about the problems in health care, they think about them, and they have opinions that may be quite useful in trying to improve conditions for the patients or clients, for themselves and their coworkers, and for their organizations. Behavioral management techniques should be employed to bring these ideas out. It will take time and effort, especially because many will not be used to being asked their opinions and because they may be reluctant to discuss their ideas in front of others (especially managers). But I believe it will be worth the time and effort.

CONTEMPORANEOUS THEORIES

Because so many areas were not addressed by the classicalists or the behavioralists, a third school of management, or motivational thought, has

 Building Comprehension Exercise begins on following page

BUILDING COMPREHENSION EXERCISE 9–3

Applying Herzberg's Theory of Motivation

Does Herzberg's theory of motivation apply to you? Do his factors motivate you, or do they just get you to move? Complete the table below as it relates to your work in your chosen health-care profession.

	Explain/give examples of this in your profession	Motivates you (explain how)	Only gets you to move (explain why)
Money	I chose OTA because of Job security + a decent salary	A decent salary will allow me to be able to get on my feet and my own home.	
Benefits	Many careers w/in OTA have great benefits	Now that insurance is required I hope to obtain a career that offers a nice package.	
Quality of the supervisor	I'm hoping as an OTA, I will work c my supervisor nicely		I may have days when we clash, but it's not going to change my mind on my career choice
Working conditions	Depending on the type of work I'll be in, it may be tough.		luckily this path offers many alternative options if one place doesn't work out.
Work rules	In the health field I will need to follow strict rules		As long as I enjoy and am successful, these rules won't bother me.
Seniority policy/benefits	Not sure what types I will get.		we'll see if it happens

Exercise continues on following page ❧ ❧ ❧

	Explain/give examples of this in your profession	*Motivates you (explain how)*	*Only gets you to move (explain why)*
Achievement	OTA is a career that offers alot of room for success + improvement.	I always want to be better and successful. I want to be great at my job	
Recognition	- Going home at night knowing that the person is that much better and appreciates you.	This will help me improve and be successful	
Responsibility	I will be responsible for the person's safety and well-being.		It's part of the job.
Advancement	OTA's have a lot of opportunities & CEUS.	I want to live well + happy so advancing is ideal	
Growth	Growth with the career + the clients	I'd like to be a part of something.	
Work itself	Challenging so different depending on location		I do what I can for success

End of exercise. Text continues on following page.

emerged. This new school of thought has led to motivational theories that can coexist with either one or both of the major paradigms. I have chosen the word *contemporaneous,* meaning "living or occurring at the same time," and its reference to facts or events, to represent this group of theories (Table 9–5).

Reinforcement Theory

You may be familiar with the basic principles of reinforcement theory from an introductory psychology class. This is a derivative of the theories of B. F. Skinner. Skinner's study of behavior modification led him to conclude that people do only what they are reinforced to do. This motivation could come in the form of *positive reinforcement,* or a reward, for performing the desired activity. Or it could be *negative reinforcement*—that is, withholding a reward when the desired activity is not performed. A third possibility is punishment. *Punishment* consists of an unpleasant consequence for not performing a certain behavior. According to Skinnerian theory, everything people do is because they are reinforced to perform that behavior. People may do what others want them to do to receive

pay or recognition. Or they do what others do *not* want just to receive attention—even if it means being reprimanded. Or people may follow rules because they do not want to face the consequences of breaking them.

Reinforcement theory certainly has a place in motivating people. No one could continue to work if he or she received nothing from a job. *Nothing* does not refer to only money, however. Millions of people volunteer their services every year. Although they receive no money, they must receive something—recognition, respect, some good feeling—or they would not continue to do it. But Skinnerian theory must be missing something also. Humans are too complex for us to say that if the right reinforcer is found, they can be trained to do exactly what is desired, and if administered correctly, they will eventually do it for no reinforcement.

However, this is essentially what Skinner[29] said in *Beyond Freedom and Dignity.* If people are trained through reinforcement, eventually the reinforcer will not have to be given every time to guarantee performance. For example, let us say a medical technologist receives a piece rate for each blood sample tested. Also assume that he or she is given the reinforcement immediately after completing

TABLE 9–5 • CONTEMPORANEOUS THEORIES OF MOTIVATION (CAN BE USED IN CONJUNCTION WITH OTHER THEORIES)

Reinforcement theory	People act because they are reinforced or rewarded to do so. To produce a behavior, one must encourage or reward that behavior. To stop (extinguish) a behavior, one must punish or ignore that behavior.
Expectancy theory	For someone to be motivated by a reward, the person must (1) want the reward and (2) believe he or she has a chance to earn or receive it.
Equity theory	People compare what they give to a job to what they receive, and they compare their giving-receiving ratio to others' giving-receiving ratios. If both cases are equal, they are satisfied. If they are giving more than they are receiving or more than others are giving, they feel the organization owes them. If they are receiving more than others are receiving, they feel guilty and work harder to establish equity.
Intrinsic-extrinsic theory	Some people are motivated through internal (intrinsic) ways that cannot be reached. People can still be motivated through one of five external (extrinsic) methods.
Level of concern	Holding people accountable for some behavior. If something is being measured, people's level of concern about that thing will be increased and they will concentrate on doing whatever it is.
Success	People are motivated to do things they are successful at; people do not do things they do poorly. This success factor can be suspended when people are learning something, if they see progress.
Interest	People are motivated to do things that are interesting; they are not motivated to do tasks that bore them.
Feedback	People need to know if they are doing well or doing poorly in order to be motivated.
Feeling tones:	The way in which someone is asked or told to perform a task. There are three tones:
Positive tone	Being asked to do something. Has the highest motivational effect.
Negative tone	Being ordered to do something. Has the second highest motivational effect; some people will do it to spite the one giving the orders, but it is a distant second.
Neutral tone	Stating that there is something to be done. Neither motivates nor demotivates.

the test. According to Skinner, after a time the pay could be withheld. The technologist completes a test and receives pay: test–pay, test–pay, test–pay, test– (nothing). Skinner's theory says that the behavior has become ingrained in the medical technologist. After not getting paid, he or she performs another test, and is then paid. However, every once in a while the pay is skipped. Then the interval between payments is increased so that two, three, four, or more tests are done before payment is again given. Skinner said this person will nevertheless keep working and that eventually he or she will be trained to produce much for little or no pay. Although gambling follows a similar scenario (except the payoffs are much less frequent), I am convinced that the first time most people completed work and did not receive pay would also be the last. To use pay as the withheld reinforcer on a regular basis would not work. Even though withholding reinforcement worked with Skinner's pigeon test subjects, it would not work with employees because people, with few exceptions, are not the same.[30]

Expectancy Theory

Developed by Victor Vroom,[31] and rather complex in the original form, expectancy theory asks two basic questions, which are diagrammed in Figure 9–1. Essentially, Vroom says that for *anything* to be motivational, the person who is to be motivated must want what is being offered and must *believe* he or she has a chance to earn it.[32] Note that in the second part of the theory it does not matter if the person actually has a chance at earning the reward—only what the person *believes* is important. The manager can be perfectly fair and equitable in these matters, but if the managee believes he or she is not capable of earning the reward, it will not be motivational. Note also that expectancy theory can be used in conjunction

with any other motivation theory.[33] Whether it is money offered by a classical manager or recognition offered by a behavioral manager, expectancy theory still applies.

As an example of expectancy, assume that training in a second health profession is a reward being offered by your employer. The first question to be asked is: "Is training in a second health profession something you desire?" If not, then you will not be motivated to perform actions that would earn you this reward. An incentive system featuring this reward would fail for you. If it is something you desire, then the second question needs to be asked: "Do you believe you have a chance of receiving the opportunity to learn a second health profession?" If you believe there is too much competition from your coworkers for the reward or that your coworkers are better qualified, this incentive plan will fail to motivate you. You will be motivated only if the reward is something you want and something you believe you have a chance to receive.[34]

Equity Theory

Equity theory is another motivator that can exist in conjunction with other motivation theories. It says that individuals will examine those things that they receive from a job—pay, recognition, respect, status, and so on—and make an internal and an external comparison (Fig. 9–2).[35] The internal comparison will involve the reward and the effort used in getting the reward. Three possibilities exist. The reward will be perceived to be less than you deserve, given the effort required. Here you will feel that you are "owed" something. Working less hard in the future may be how you even the score. At the opposite extreme, the reward may outweigh the effort. Here the theory says you will feel guilty about receiving more than you deserved. The third possibility is that the two

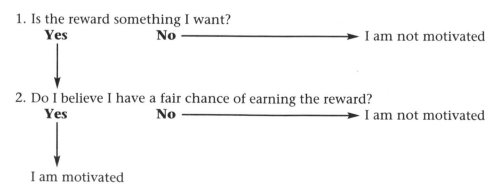

FIGURE 9–1 • Expectancy theory asks these two basic questions. It can be used with any reward and with any other motivation theory.

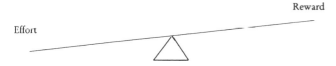

FIGURE 9–2 • The balance between effort and reward. In this example, the person will feel something is owed to him or her.

are perceived as being equal and you are relatively satisfied.[36]

The external comparison involves a person's comparing his or her internal reward-effort ratio to the perceived reward-effort ratios of others. Again, three possibilities exist. You may perceive that a coworker's ratio is higher than your own (the coworker received more for his or her efforts than you did). This may also lead to the feeling that you are owed something. Second, you may perceive that a coworker's ratio is lower than yours (the coworker received less for his or her efforts than you did). In this case the theory says you will feel guilty and will work harder to justify to yourself the receiving of greater rewards. The third possibility is that the ratios will be perceived as equal and fairness has prevailed.[37]

Equity theory does not provide a means to directly motivate people. Instead, like expectancy theory, it attempts to demonstrate that motivation is a complex endeavor. The theory appears to be valid based only on personal experiences of noting how often people are concerned about how much (or how little) their coworkers are working.

Intrinsic-Extrinsic Theory

The final theory to be discussed here comes from Madeline Hunter of the University of California, Los Angeles. Hunter believes that there is *intrinsic motivation* (internal) and *extrinsic motivation* (external). She believes that internal motivation, that from within each person, cannot be directly manipulated. She believes that a person can be motivated only by influencing external factors. She lists five external factors for motivating:

1. Level of concern
2. Feedback
3. Success
4. Interest
5. Feeling tone

Level of concern involves accountability. If you are going to be held accountable for something, you will be concerned about it and motivated to act on that concern. For example, a new manager has a reputation for demanding punctuality. Your entire merit raise depends on your getting to work on time. Because you will be held accountable, you are motivated to be at work on time. If the manager did not care, you probably would not either. Or think of a class where a teacher said that you would not be tested on some of the material. Unless another of these extrinsic factors applied (or you possessed intrinsic motivation), you would not be motivated to learn that material. If the teacher were to say, however, that this same material would be half of the next exam, you probably would sit up and take notice. (Notice how expectancy theory can come into play here. You also have to want the merit raise or want to and expect that you can do well on the exam to be motivated.)

Feedback can motivate you if it is timely and accurate. If you know how well you are doing, Hunter says you are motivated to keep doing it. Conversely, if you have no idea of how you are performing, you will not be as motivated to continue. As an example, how long would you continue to play a game if you never knew the score? How would you know if you were doing well or poorly? Or, how motivational is an annual performance review? If you are only told once a year that you are doing well, it is unlikely that you are being motivated by this feedback.

Success as a motivator is connected to feedback. If you are successful at something, you are motivated to continue doing it—of course, you may need feedback to know whether or not you are doing well. On the other hand, if you are not good at something, you are not motivated to continue. This success factor does not apply to the learning phase, though. The length of the learning phase during which people will tolerate poor performance is limited and variable, but if progress is being made, most people will continue to try. Again, feedback from others may be vital to know that improvement is being made. This is especially true when the tasks are complex and progress is slow.

Success and feedback certainly appear to apply to learning within a health profession. If someone tried to learn the material in an entire health profession in one unbroken 2-, 3-, or 4-year program, he or she would see little progress (success) and little feedback. By dividing the material into separate classes or units, a person can see progress (completing each term's classes or units) and receive feedback (class or unit grades) in smaller increments. Hunter's theory states that this success and feedback cycle is also required when learning a new job skill or simply when adapting to a new work environment.

Interest in an activity is also motivating. Job rotation, job enlargement, and job enrichment are all attempts at keeping work interesting. Interest can also be maintained through social contacts at work, through an interesting physical work environment, and from challenging work that provides a learning experience. Here you can see how information presented in previous chapters fits together in the complex entity called the "working environment."

The fifth factor in Hunter's theory is *feeling tone;* that is, the way in which communications between the manager and managee are handled. Hunter says there are three feeling tones—positive, negative, and neutral. A *positive feeling tone* includes being asked to perform a task: "Would you please take this next patient?" Even if there is no real choice, if a manager *asks* someone to take a patient to another department, the person will usually feel better about it than if a negative tone is used. A *negative tone* means someone is being commanded to do something, especially in an unpleasant way: "Get this next patient. Now." This is motivating—through fear, intimidation, and use of institutional power (power from having a position of authority in the institution), but it is a distant second to positive tone. Also a negative feeling tone is not effective with men. As mentioned in Chapter 3, research by Dr. Deborah Tannen[38] has shown that men, because they live in a hierarchical world, are much less likely to respond to commanding, negative feeling tone. Finally, *neutral feeling tone* is neither positive nor negative; it is simply a statement of fact without sarcastic, commanding, or other tones. An example is the statement, "Another patient is here." Neutral feeling tone does not demotivate, but it does not motivate either.

A Manager's View

Why do managers follow some of these theories and not others? There are actually a number of reasons. Some managers believe in a certain system. Their upbringing and personal, premanagement experiences tell them that a certain method is correct. Some managers were educated, formally or informally, in a certain method. Others have had no training and have had to employ their own methods. These may resemble those of one of the established systems. Many managers may believe in one method or another but use that of their boss or of the organization. Also, sometimes the managees force, or allow, a manager to adopt a particular method.

This last reason is of most concern here. The people in a department may cause a manager to use particular tactics. For example, if a department

is cohesive, supportive, and responsive, a manager will be able to apply many of the behavioral methods. Behavioral methods rely on good relations between manager and managee. They also require the *participation* of the managees. Conversely, if the managees refuse to participate, behavioral methods fail, possibly forcing the manager to employ classical methods.

There may also be individual differences. A manager may use behavioral methods on all but one person in a department if that person fails to respond to those methods. Behavioral methods generally depend on managees' taking responsibility for their work and earning the manager's trust. Responsibility for completing the work means completing it at a high level of quality and efficiency without a large amount of supervision. Some people cannot, or will not, make this commitment. They may try to take advantage of the system and do much less than their share. They should not be surprised, then, when the manager employs some of the restrictive, close supervision ideals of the classical writers. Also, the manager must trust the managee to work independently. Trust takes time to earn; the managee must first demonstrate that he or she can be depended on before autonomy is granted. Managees who do not take the time and do not make the effort to earn a manager's trust should not be surprised if they are treated differently from those who have proven themselves.

Possibly the most difficult aspects of behavioralism for many managers to overcome are those of power loss and invested effort. Using behavioralism requires that the manager relinquish some power. It is transferred to the managees so that they may self-supervise, self-check, self-schedule, or make decisions on their own. Sometimes the choices made are not the same as the manager would have made, and this is difficult for some bosses.

The second potential problem is the amount of effort a manager must invest to start and maintain a more behavioral working environment. It takes much more effort and patience to use behavioral methods than classical ones. Behavioral management concerns teams, groups, individual feelings, and so on. Classical motivation is more objective and concrete. It takes time to find each person's level on Maslow's hierarchy or to try to ensure that every position contains learning experiences. Because of this, some managers, already pressed for time, may elect not to employ many or any behavioral techniques.

Finally, one of the difficult jobs for any manager is trying to find motivational techniques that will

 Building Comprehension Exercise begins on following page

BUILDING COMPREHENSION EXERCISE 9–4

Identifying External Motivators

Which of Madeline Hunter's external factors would motivate you? Give examples of each factor and explain why it motivates you.

	Motivates Me	*Example*	*Why It Motivates Me*
Level of concern	Being accountable for my Job + actions	Being on time to work	It sets a good example. It shows how serious + motivated I am to be here.
Feedback	Discussing my Job	a review talking i on my performance.	I would like to know if I'm making errors otherwise I may never resolve it.
Success	Doing my Job well	Progress and feed back lead to success	I want to be great at what I will be doing.
Interest	enjoying my career	Choosing activities that are enjoyable	the best success comes when client + COTA are interested in activities
Feeling tone	Positive feeling tone	" would you please take this to the next client "	Having this positive relationship lowers stress + creates a positive environment.

End of exercise. Text continues on following page.

work. By now it should be apparent by the number of theories that exist that there is no consensus as to what works. Here, informed managees may be able to help their managers and themselves.

A Managee's View

Most people wait to be motivated. This is not the best way to get what you want. Waiting to be motivated by a manager who may not have the time, interest, or ability to discern what will motivate you should be too random of an experience to satisfy you. Because you have a direct interest in being motivated to work, you should not only participate in the process, you should take the lead. And you do have an interest in being motivated because being motivated means not only that you want to work, but also that you want to improve, excel, and even look forward to work. This may be the difference between "working" and "having a career." The question now is how to proceed, and this is depicted in Figure 9–3.

The first step should be for you to apply the theories in this chapter to yourself. Analyze your needs. Discover what it is that you want. Ask your-

self, "What will motivate me?" You must know what you want before you can go after it.

Second, find out whether or not your needs can be fulfilled at work. If not, find out where they can be met. If they can be met at work, then find out which existing motivators can apply toward you. If none of the existing work motivators applies to you, create some that will.

Third, approach your manager. Remember that you both have an interest in your being motivated to work. Of course it will be easier for you to ask to apply existing motivators to your situation. If you are asking for something different, make sure that you:

1. Outline the benefits to your patients or clients.
2. Outline the benefits to your employer.
3. Outline the benefits to yourself.
4. Explain everything in a logical, rational manner.

Make your proposal so sensible and compelling that it will be difficult for the manager to refuse.

Fourth, remember to be honest with yourself about what you want and, if necessary, be creative in how your employer can use this to motivate you. For example, maybe you have always had an interest in financial or numerical affairs, but you are a respiratory therapist. Maybe the chance to order supplies, monitor the inventory, or complete a statistical analysis will motivate you. Even if it is only 1 to 2 hours per week, if it will keep you interested and it helps the manager or department, you may be able to convince management of the mutual benefits. The same may be true if you wish to prepare a continuing education session for the department, represent your department to other departments, or become more specialized or more generalized. The most important point is that for you to be motivated and achieve the most that you can, it is almost imperative that you take the lead. If you do not know what will motivate you, how can anyone else?

Summary

The major motivational theorists have been presented along with the views of their theories from managers' and a managees' perspectives. This information can be useful before as well as after a job has been obtained. Before accepting a position, it may help if you analyze the type of motivational theory you feel would work best for you. It will help your analysis and learning of the material for

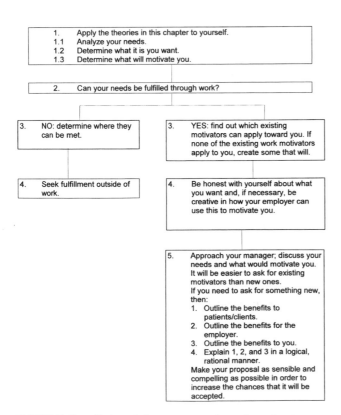

FIGURE 9–3 • Determining your needs and motivation toward meeting those needs.

 Building Comprehension Exercise begins on following page

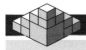

BUILDING COMPREHENSION EXERCISE 9–5

What Motivates You?

Part 1

For each of the following factors, mark the motivation level that applies to you (e.g., highly motivating, somewhat motivating, or not motivating). Then rank the factors from 1 to 20, with 1 being the factor that motivates you the most.

Rank		Highly Motivating	Somewhat Motivating	Not Motivating
___	1. Money (salary)	_____	_____	_____
___	2. Piece-rate pay	_____	_____	_____
___	3. Desire to help others	_____	_____	_____
___	4. Annual raise	_____	_____	_____
___	5. Paid health insurance	_____	_____	_____
___	6. Paid life insurance	_____	_____	_____
___	7. Status job title	_____	_____	_____
___	8. Learning on the job	_____	_____	_____
___	9. Achievement	_____	_____	_____
___	10. Promotions	_____	_____	_____
___	11. Recognition	_____	_____	_____
___	12. Feedback	_____	_____	_____
___	13. Success	_____	_____	_____
___	14. Responsibility	_____	_____	_____
___	15. Autonomy	_____	_____	_____
___	16. Setting own goals	_____	_____	_____
___	17. Interesting work	_____	_____	_____
___	18. Positive feeling tone	_____	_____	_____
___	19. Being held accountable	_____	_____	_____
___	20. A deadline	_____	_____	_____

Exercise continues on following page ❖ ❖ ❖

Part 2

Explain your results and discuss how you would want a manager to motivate you.

_____

_____

_____

_____

_____

End of exercises. Text continues on following page.

you to make a list of the aspects and assumptions of the major categories. This is especially true of the behavioral and classical theories. Decide which is best for you. Then, during a job interview, look for evidence that points to the methods used by the manager. Classify each employer, and try to obtain the best match between your needs and the methods of the organization.

Once you have taken a job, use the information in this chapter to choose the motivators that you feel will work best applied to you. Last, do not forget that your actions can influence the methods your manager selects. If he or she asks for your opinion or attempts team building, and so on, do what you can to cooperate. This is similar to the decision-making situation. If you are asked and do not respond, do not be surprised if you are never asked again.

REFERENCES

1. Daft, RL: Management, ed 5. Dryden, Fort Worth, 2000, p. 51.
2. Kreitner, R: Management, ed 4. Houghton Mifflin, Boston, 1989, pp 57–59, 72–73.
3. Daft, pp 62–63.
4. Draft, p 537.
5. Stevenson, W: Production Operations Management, ed 6. Irwin/McGraw-Hill, Boston, 1999, p 20.
6. Gini, AR, and Sullivan, TJ: It Comes with the Territory. Random House, New York, 1989, pp 41–49.
7. Etzioni, A: Modern Organizations. Prentice-Hall, Englewood Cliffs, NJ, 1964, p 21.
8. Dilworth, J: Operations Management, ed 3. Dryden, Fort Worth, 2000, p 26.
9. Stevenson, p 23.
10. Stevenson, p 20.
11. Daft, pp 46–47.
12. Draft, p 50.
13. Draft, p 49.
14. Draft, p 63.
15. Draft, pp 51–52.
16. Kreitner, pp 68–70.
17. Mondy, RW, et al: Management: Concepts, Practices, and Skills. Allyn and Bacon, Boston, 1991, pp 293–95.
18. Aldag, RJ, and Stearns, TM: Management. Southwestern Publishing, Cincinnati, 1991, pp 453–54.
19. Mondy, pp 294–95.
20. Daft, p 539.
21. Draft, p 540.
22. Mondy, pp 298–304.
23. Van Fleet, DD: Contemporary Management, ed 3. Houghton Mifflin, Boston, 1993, pp 356–57.
24. Daft, p 541.
25. Draft, p 563.
26. Mondy, pp 300–303.
27. Van Fleet, p 357.
28. Scott, WR: Organizations: Rational, Natural, and Open Systems, ed 2. Prentice-Hall, Englewood Cliffs, NJ, 1987, p 87.
29. Daft, p 563.
30. Van Fleet, 367–70.
31. Daft, p 545–47.
32. Kreitner, pp 436–38.
33. Mondy, pp 309–11.
34. Van Fleet, pp 361–62.
35. Aldag, and Stearns, pp 421–26.
36. Mondy, pp 306–07.
37. Van Fleet, pp 364–65.
38. Tannen, D: You Just Don't Understand. Ballantine, New York, 1990, p 43.

10 · Change

Objectives

On completion of this chapter, the reader will be able to:

☐ Identify and define the ways people show resistance to change.

☐ Identify and define the causes of resistance to change.

☐ Identify and explain how change is accomplished.

☐ Explain the importance of knowing how to identify resistance to change, causes of resistance to change, and how change is accomplished.

☐ Identify methods of coping with change.

☐ Explain the importance of being able to accept and cope with change.

Western cultures have only one constant feature—change.[1] That things change, improve, and progress is the basis for our system and is so inherent that it is taken for granted. Yet most people resist change. We want change, we work for change, but we cling to traditions and the old way of doing things. This chapter explores the dynamics of change and how it is resisted and why; it also offers coping strategies. However, simply realizing and acknowledging that we do resist change and understanding why we resist it should provide some improvement in our ability to handle change and increase our acceptance of it.

That change is an important topic for health professions is indisputable. Examine this brief list of major recent changes in the health industry and in health technology:

- Managed care
- AIDS and universal precautions
- Changes in reimbursement methods
- Concerns with the increasing costs of health care

- The aging of the population
- Magnetic resonance imaging (MRI) scanners
- Increased competition among health-care providers
- Diagnosis-related groups (DRGs)
- Use of computers
- Automated lab testing

Of course, there are many other changes in health care and in daily life that could be listed. Despite these changes and despite change being an integral part of our society, many people are reluctant to change and resist change.

This chapter examines how resistance to change in general is demonstrated, ranging from simple to drastic responses. The underlying causes for resistance to change is discussed. The methods by which many changes are brought about are explained. Finally, methods for coping with change are presented.

How Resistance to Change Is Shown

Resistance to change can be demonstrated through many different behaviors, as listed in Figure 10–1. Some responses are relatively simple, and although they may be annoying, their effect is less severe. Other reactions are more complex and more drastic. The consequences of these reactions can be much more significant for the managee, as well as the manager.

I have identified six general ways in which people show resistance to change in the working environment. They are:

1. Regression
2. Lower productivity
3. Sabotage
4. Absenteeism
5. Transfer
6. Resignation

Each is explained, and the effects of each discussed.

Regression is one of the simpler responses to change. People who dislike a particular change may regress to a state in which they pretend not to know how to perform all or part of their jobs.[2] Their basic thought is, "If you are going to change the rules, fine. Then you will not only have to tell me how to do things the new way, but you will have to tell me how to do everything." For example, most therapies or diagnostic procedures follow a basic format. If one routine is changed, a person resisting through regression will suddenly begin to ask for instructions on how to perform all the procedures. Regression is a rather mild form of opposing change, even if it is annoying and childlike.

Lower productivity is a method of showing resistance to change, and the intention is to have the change reversed. In this method people deliberately reduce their work output.[3] Their hope is that they will not be caught and that the manager will believe that the decrease in productivity is due to

the change. Therefore, the change will be eliminated and things will return to the way they were before.

A much more severe response to change, and one that may also be an attempt to have the change repealed, is sabotage.[4] *Sabotage* is a deliberate action meant to harm the organization. The sabotage may be subtle; for instance, when a patient's or client's billing paperwork is deliberately discarded. This action may hurt the employer, but it may also go undetected. It then has no effect on reversing the change, and ultimately, the lost revenue damages not only the employer but the employee as well. (What's bad for the company is bad for the workers.) Most people who engage in sabotage do not see it this way, however. They often view it as justifiable revenge. Other forms of sabotage include mislaying equipment, wasting supplies, and making patients delay their appointments—scheduling them for a later date, or canceling appointments and rescheduling them for later. Some workers have gone so far as to deliberately break medical equipment, some of which costs thousands of dollars to replace and repair. Although these actions are severe, they occur far more often than one would initially suspect.

The last three methods of showing resistance to change are all attempts to escape change. They range from milder to more severe forms of escape and include absenteeism, transfer, and resignation.

Absenteeism can include tardiness; calling in sick when one is not (and usually being compensated for staying home); returning late from lunch or breaks; taking frequent bathroom, cigarette, or other breaks; or missing work (with no compensation).[5] Absenteeism is a way in which people avoid facing both the change and their dislike of the change. It fails to resolve the situation because the person delays accepting the changed situation and also delays trying to cope with it. However, absenteeism is a more complex symptom than this because problems other than change can cause one to be late for or miss work. Although missing work may affect the employer or place an extra burden on other employees, it may also be minimal, depending on the situation. However, there is also a burden on the person who is absent. The unresolved conflict that the person is trying to escape can take a greater toll and have a more deleterious effect than would learning to cope with the change.

Requesting a *transfer* to another department in the organization is another means of escape that can be triggered by change or by other factors.[6] This response is more complicated or more involved and often has fewer negative aspects. In addition to being an escape response, transferring

Less severe		More severe
Regression	Lower Productivity	Sabotage
Absenteeism	Transfer	Resignation

FIGURE 10–1 • Resistance to change can be demonstrated through many different behaviors. Some are relatively simple responses, and although annoying, create effects that are not too severe. Other reactions are more complex and drastic.

might also be considered a coping strategy by some. One person may be overreacting to change by escaping through transfer. To someone else to whom the change (possibly a "negative" change) is truly unbearable, transferring may be a way of coping. The person has dealt with change by leaving the area but not the organization. Of course, this avenue is not open to everyone because there may not be a position to transfer to or the person may not have the necessary training to enter another health profession.

Finally, the most extreme form of escape, and the one having the greatest impact on the managee, is *resignation*.[7] Like transferring, leaving the organization might be escape to some or coping to others. However, the negative effects on the employee can be great. It may be difficult to find another job, and when one is found, it may be for less remuneration and with less seniority. When quitting is an impulse, an overreaction, or an act of revenge, it is almost always more punishing to the employee than to the employer—few employers consider people irreplaceable. But if the situation is truly unbearable and transferring is not possible, it may be the only option left. However, you should always try to cope with and manage the situation through other methods before making such a drastic move. When resignation is the answer, it should always be planned and thought through in a logical, rational manner after all other possibilities have been tried and failed.

Causes of Resistance to Change

The different ways in which people resist change have been presented. Now the causes of resistance will be examined. There are at least 10 different causes that have been identified. They are briefly described in Table 10–1, and they include:

1. Fear
2. Inertia
3. Inconvenience
4. Economics
5. Surprise
6. Threats to the informal organization
7. Revenge
8. Misunderstanding
9. Poor timing
10. Poor approach

Generally, those at the top of this list are more prevalent or more powerful causes of resistance to change.

Fear includes fear of failure, fear of the unknown, and general uncertainty.[8] Fear is a major reason people resist change. The old situation is known, and people are much more comfortable with what they know than what they don't. In fact, humanity's greatest fear may be fear of the unknown. Change brings about questions and

TABLE 10–1 • CAUSES OF RESISTANCE TO CHANGE

Fear	The change or the effects of the change are unknown, and people are afraid of what they don't know.
Inertia	The old ways have momentum that sustains them; change must not only gain its own momentum but must also stop that of the old method.
Inconvenience	Change requires effort, and some people do not want to be bothered with putting forth any additional effort.
Economics	The change has or it is thought to have a negative financial effect.
Surprise	The change has come about without warning.
Threats to the informal organization	The social order, work groups, or cliques will be, in the managees' view, adversely affected.
Revenge	People want to retaliate for a previous event.
Misunderstanding	The change was not clear to understand, or the managees did not grasp the concept or were mistaken as to the effects of the change.
Poor timing	The change coincided poorly with other events.
Poor approach	The method for accomplishing the change was inappropriate or incorrect.

Note: Generally, those reactions at the top of this list are more prevalent or more powerful causes of resistance to change.

 Building Comprehension Exercise begins on following page

BUILDING COMPREHENSION EXERCISE 10–1

Evaluating Resistance to Change

Which of the ways people show resistance to change have you used, and which have you seen others use? Describe the incidents. What, if anything, do you think the organization could have done to prevent or significantly reduce the resistance?

	I used:	Others used:	Describe the incident.
Regression			

How I think the resistance could have been reduced:

Lower productivity			

How I think the resistance could have been reduced:

Sabotage			

How I think the resistance could have been reduced:

Exercise continues on following page ⬙ ⬙ ⬙

	I used:	*Others used:*	*Describe the incident.*
Absenteeism			

How I think the
resistance could
have been reduced:

	I used:	*Others used:*	*Describe the incident.*
Transfer			

How I think the
resistance could
have been reduced:

	I used:	*Others used:*	*Describe the incident.*
Resignation			

How I think the
resistance could
have been reduced:

End of exercise. Text continues on following page.

uncertainty. Because work is such a large part of one's life, uncertainty is often unwelcome. Although any reaction to this fear is possible, it is probably more common for people to use absenteeism, transfer, sabotage, and possibly resignation, rather than regression, as a coping mechanism.

Inertia is another major means of resisting change.[9] *Inertia* is the tendency of a moving object to continue moving, and the tendency of an object at rest to remain at rest. Both halves of the definition might apply here, but the first half is especially true. Organizations, policies, and procedures have momentum. They move and their inertia takes over. So, organizations, policies, and procedures that are in place and moving tend to remain in place, moving, and in force.[10] They take on lives of their own. Efforts to implement change do not face only the problem of getting started, of building their own inertia but also the problem of counteracting the inertia of previous policies. The concept of inertia also manifests in common wisdom such as, "That's the way we've always done it" and "If it's not broken, don't fix it." These maxims represent the idea that current practice should remain in force and unchanged. That there is resistance to change can be considered further evidence of the inertia principle in organizations.

The next factor, *inconvenience,* may be related to inertia. Some people resist change because it is inconvenient for them to alter the way they do things.[11] Maybe the reason the old ways have inertia is because it is inconvenient for people to learn new ways. Change, by its very nature, requires difference from the past. For people to change, they must delete something from the past and learn something new—a procedure, charting, billing, or scheduling method, or how to operate a new piece of equipment. Many people regard learning as work. It takes effort and practice. It would be much more convenient to continue in the old manner and forget about the changes.

For certain situations the main motive for resisting change may be *economics.* Changes brought about by automation may foster resistance because people fear that their jobs will be lost to a machine.[12] This is a genuine concern as has been seen in health-care laboratories. The need for medical technologists has decreased as machines like the SMA-12 perform more and more of the lab work. In general, medical fields will remain rather labor intensive for the foreseeable future. However, automation is not the only factor that may cause resistance to change because of economic concerns.

There is a very real concern about the cost of health care in the United States. Many hospitals and health facilities have had to close because of economic pressure from increased competition and from cost-payment control methods of government and other third-party payers. Although many health professions are in need of additional workers, there is local concern for facilities in poor areas. On the other hand, the population is aging, and the labor pool is getting smaller. Both factors create higher demand for health-care professionals.

Another aspect of economics as a cause of resistance to change is the impact on personnel within a department. A new worker may threaten those with more seniority if it is believed that the new person is more likely to receive a promotion. Or a new manager may have a different opinion of merit raises and promotions that affect the plans of those who were there first. For these reasons, employees may resist accepting or working with the new worker, or they may resist the new manager's methods.

When change takes people by *surprise,* they usually resist more than if the change is introduced gradually.[13] It is also readily apparent that a person taken by surprise by a change was not involved in the change decision. Generally, change is better accepted when the people affected by it are involved.[14]

Social connections are an integral part of work. Many changes are resisted because they *threaten the informal organization* and the social relations within.[15] People and groups expend considerable energy in building these relations and in establishing status and a group hierarchy. When these are threatened by change, many people, who have a vested interest in the current group, will resist to avoid losing their positions.[16] They may also resist the change to avoid having to expend additional energy to establish new associations. Although the impetus for the resistance may come from subconscious sources, the sources are still real and compelling.

Revenge can be a motive for resisting change.[17] This reaction may come about when managees dislike a manager or when they feel they have been wronged by the organization. The managees may feel that sabotaging the change effort may even the score between themselves and the manager or organization.

Misunderstanding the change may cause opposition.[18] The intent of the change may not be understood. Possibly the motive behind the change has been assumed—and assumed incorrectly. Or the ultimate goal of the change has been presented in a confusing way. Whatever the situation, there has been a lack of communication, and it is difficult to cooperate with something you don't understand.[19]

Poor timing of a change may cause increased resistance.[20] For example, reducing workers' hours at the same time that inflation is pushing up prices may cause greater than normal resistance. Or a change in starting time may come just as someone's child begins school, making it impossible for the parent to bring the child to school. So the poor timing may be related to some other factor on the job, or it may be totally unrelated to work. The effect can still be the same.

Finally, resistance to change can be increased or decreased to a certain degree by the way the change is presented. A *poor approach* to the explanation for why the change is occurring may increase the resistance.[21] A tactful and sensitive approach may be required, or it may be better to discuss the change in private.

How Change Is Accomplished

Change is accomplished in different ways depending on the style of the manager or the style of the manager's manager, and on the situation that needs changing. The common methods that I have identified are summarized in Table 10–2 and include:

- Training
- Directive
- Participative decision making
- Manipulation
- Trial period
- New-person method

Small changes may be accomplished in a short training session or by directive. Moderate changes may be made through training, by directive, through participative methods, by manipulation, or by trial period. Large-scale changes can be made through training, by directive, through participative methods, by manipulation, by trial period, or by the new-person method. Often, the new-person method is favored for major changes.

The method that generally receives the most attention in management circles is *training*. Using training to bring about change is a simple concept to explain. The change is actually brought about by training people in new methods or techniques.[22] The change occurs almost simultaneously with the learning and implementation of the new ways, and the act of changing is almost transparent to the worker. Although this may seem obvious when training is for new job skills (using a new skill, by definition, means that something is changed, or else it can't be new), sometimes organizational change is integrated with new learning. For example, introducing a new, more centralized word processing system may be a way of also introducing organizational change. If the former system was decentralized with six locations and six independent managers, a centralized system might also allow for a reduction in the

TABLE 10–2 • DIFFERENT WAYS TO ACCOMPLISH CHANGE

Change Method	Summary	Type of Change the Method Is Used for
Training	Educating people on how to use a new method helps the change to the new method.	Small Moderate Large
Directive	Change is implemented by direct order; compliance is mandatory.	Small Moderate Large
Participative decision making	The exact change is not predetermined. A change will occur, but when the change will occur is decided by management and managees together.	Moderate Large
Manipulation	Procedure appears to be participative decision making, but the manager has predetermined the outcome. The manager guides the managees toward suggesting the change he or she has already decided on.	Moderate Large
Trial period	The change is tried on a temporary basis and then evaluated. It is then made permanent, altered, or discarded.	Moderate Large
New-person method	Replacing the manager or other key personnel because people will expect the new person to change things.	Large

 Building Comprehension Exercise begins on following page

BUILDING COMPREHENSION EXERCISE 10–2

Examining the Causes of Resistance to Change

Which of these causes of resistance to change have you experienced? Describe each incident.
What, if anything, could have been done to prevent this?

	I have experienced:	Describe the incident.
Fear		
How could this have been prevented?		
Inertia		
How could this have been prevented?		
Inconvenience		
How could this have been prevented?		
Economics		
How could this have been prevented?		

Exercise continues on following page 🔹🔹🔹

	I have experienced:	*Describe the incident.*
Surprise		
How could this have been prevented?		
Threats to the informal organization		
How could this have been prevented?		
Revenge		
How could this have been prevented?		
Misunderstanding		
How could this have been prevented?		

Exercise continues on following page ☙ ☙ ☙

	I have experienced:	*Describe the incident.*
Poor timing		
How could this have been prevented?		
Poor approach		
How could this have been prevented?		

End of exercise. Text continues on following page.

number or reshuffling of managers. Training and working on the new central system under fewer or different managers accomplishes two changes at the same time. And, workers go through only one disruption.

Classical, authoritarian managers are typically more prone to making change by *directive*. The decision to change, method, timing, and other factors concerning the change are all made by the manager.[23] The orders are usually in writing and posted, and sometimes require that each employee sign or initial them. It is assumed that they will be obeyed. Of course, not everyone will understand the directive. Nor will everyone obey or obey in the same way. Without checking, the change may not be made at all. Still, the use of a directive is a fairly common way for change to be attempted.

Behavioral managers are more likely to make changes by *participative decision making*. In this method the managees participate in the decision to change and in deciding the way the change will be implemented.[24] The belief is that employees can and will make valuable contributions to decision making, and that by being involved in the decision or change from the beginning, they will be more likely to accept the change. Also, the change will cause less disruption—of work processes and for the workers.

If you as a worker are involved in participative decision making and change, it is in your best interest to become involved. To do so will encourage the manager to use this method again. If you just sit there and do not contribute (as many people do in their first experiences with this method), the manager may abandon the idea as a waste of time for everyone. And you should become involved even if you are not particularly concerned about the issue. Some day there will be a change you do care about, but if the manager gave up on involving the managees, you may have little or no chance to provide your input.

Unfortunately, there are managers who want to appear to be using participative decision making, but they can't quite bring themselves to relinquish power and control to the managees. Both of these occur in true participative decision making, although the degree of control and power that is delegated can vary. Instead, some managers bring about change by *manipulation*.

As an example, let us say that the physical therapy department is going to expand its hours to better serve its clientele. This change will require rearranging working hours. A participative manager might call a meeting of all the therapists and say, "Here are the new hours. As a group, you may decide which hours you each want, as long as you

each work 40 hours per week and these times are covered." A manager using manipulation might also call a meeting. He or she may ask for ideas. The therapists might propose this or that scheme until someone suggests the schedule that the manager has already decided to use. The manager says something like, "That's a great idea; the best one yet. This is what we will use." The illusion is maintained that the managees made the change, but in reality and unknown to them, it had already been decided.[25] This manipulation may seem less risky for the manager. However, the day may come (and it usually does) when the managees find out that they were being deceived. The resultant backlash, damage, and loss of trust in the manager is a far worse consequence than that of a poor decision managees might make. It would probably be better if the manager had just made the decision by directive.

One method of accomplishing change that can be used alone or with one of the other methods is the *trial period*. It is fairly common and has some advantages. It involves making a change temporarily for a given time.[26] At the end of the period (2 weeks, 1 month, and so on), the new way is evaluated to see if it worked and how well it worked. If it failed, the old way is reinstated or another new method is tried. Managees tend to accept this method better than some other methods; however, it must be a true trial period for maximum effectiveness. If it is known that the new way will remain whether it works or not or whether it receives poor evaluations or not, this method is no better (or different) than manipulation. As a managee, if you are involved in a true trial period change, it is in your best interest to give it a fair chance and an honest evaluation. As mentioned when discussing participative decision making, giving a change a fair chance during the trial period reinforces the value of the trial-period method with the manager. This encourages him or her to value the critiques the managees provide and also to consider using the trial period again.

Possibly one of the most time-honored methods of making change is the *new-person method*. It is a rather simple idea—replace someone from the old regime with a new person to facilitate the change.[27] Commonly, it is the manager who is replaced. The concept is that people expect new managers to do things their own way.[28] This means change. As long as people expect change with a new person, getting a new person is a relatively simple means of making change. For example, let's say that upper management wants to drastically reduce or expand a department. To "ease" the change and disruption, they bring in a new manager. The department will expect changes

 Building Comprehension Exercise begins on following page

BUILDING COMPREHENSION EXERCISE 10–3

Accomplishing Change

Which methods of accomplishing change have you witnessed? What type (size) of change was trying to be accomplished? What type of resistance to this change was present? Explain each situation you witnessed.

Change Method	Size of Change	Resistance to this Change	
Training	Small	Regression	Lower productivity
	Moderate	Sabotage	Absenteeism
	Large	Transfer	Resignation
Explanation			
Directive	Small	Regression	Lower productivity
	Moderate	Sabotage	Absenteeism
	Large	Transfer	Resignation
Explanation			
Participation	Small	Regression	Lower productivity
	Moderate	Sabotage	Absenteeism
	Large	Transfer	Resignation
Explanation			

Exercise continues on following page 🔷🔷🔷

Change Method	Size of Change	Resistance to this Change	
Manipulation	Small	Regression	Lower productivity
	Moderate	Sabotage	Absenteeism
	Large	Transfer	Resignation
Explanation			
Trial period	Small	Regression	Lower productivity
	Moderate	Sabotage	Absenteeism
	Large	Transfer	Resignation
Explanation			
New-person method	Small	Regression	Lower productivity
	Moderate	Sabotage	Absenteeism
	Large	Transfer	Resignation
Explanation			

End of exercise. Text continues on following page.

anyway, so maybe it will not be much of a surprise when it actually happens. There is not a large body of research to support or disprove the effectiveness of this method, but it is relatively common even if it is harsh on the outgoing boss.

The ways in which change is resisted, the causes of resistance, and the way change is accomplished are many and varied. However, knowing the varieties is more than an academic exercise. The information can best be used when it leads to coping with change.

Coping with Change

The first decision to be made when confronted with change is whether to fight, escape, or attempt to cope with it. If a change occurs that for some reason is morally or ethically unacceptable to you, you may have to resist or consider escaping it through transfer or resignation. Because the health professions are so specialized, it may not be possible to transfer to another department. But, with more and more hospitals and other health-care organizations combining into large networks and having multiple sites, it may be possible to change locations. Depending on the situation, transferring to another work shift or switching from full-time to part-time may be viable alternatives too. However, there are times when you may feel that you have to leave the organization. In these cases it is usually best that you not quit until you have another position. It is usually easier to go from one job to another than to go from being unemployed to employed. In addition, the time required to find a new job is almost impossible to predict, so it makes more sense financially to find a new employer first.

If you will not be resisting change or escaping from it, you will probably be attempting to cope with the change. The value in learning about change is that it enables you to better cope with it. In resisting change, you expend energy that might be better used elsewhere, and you stress yourself unnecessarily. Often, people become enraged, excited, or agitated over a change—to no effect. The change does not go away, and the manager (often the focus of the agitation) remains unaffected, either because he or she does not know you are upset, does not care, or is unable to alter the change. Therefore, all that is accomplished in some cases is that you become disquieted and disturbed; but nothing changes. Your body systems are put on alert, but the change is still occurring and the manager may be oblivious. You can arrive at an approximation of your tendency to cope with or resist change by answering the questions in Building Comprehension Exercise 10–4. If a change is inevitable—for example, in the case of corporate merger, coworker retirement, equipment modernization—it is far healthier to accept it rather than uselessly resist it (see Chap. 12 on the subject of stress). At these and other times, you may need a coping strategy.

SPECIFIC STRATEGIES

There are six strategies that can be employed when trying to cope with change. These include acceptance, participation, learning, utilization, support and assistance, and negotiation (Table 10–3).

First, try simply to *accept the change*. For many people, accepting change may not be simple. Many people, when confronted with something new, immediately set about listing all the negative aspects about it.[29] Frequently the first thing mentioned is that the new way is not the old way (stating the obvious does not deter some individuals). To accept and cope with change, these people and others should look for the good in the change.

TABLE 10–3 • SIX STRATEGIES THAT MANAGEES MAY USE FOR COPING WITH CHANGE

Coping Strategies for Change	Definition
Acceptance	Look for positive aspects.
Participation	Take part in the change.
Learning	Become thoroughly familiar with the change.
Utilization	Implement the change; use it.
Support and Assistance	Learn and utilize the change and teach it to others.
Negotiation	Arrange for an alteration to part of the change.

 Building Comprehension Exercise begins on following page

Assessing Your Feelings toward Change

Evaluate your agreement with the following statements. (SA=Strongly Agree, A=Agree, U=Unsure, D=Disagree, SD=Strongly Disagree)

	SA	A	U	D	SD
1. For me, change is an opportunity.					
2. If new equipment were purchased at work, I would want to be one of the first to learn all about it.					
3. I like variety.					
4. I adapt to changes quickly.					
5. When it comes to change, I am confident that I can adapt.					
6. If my department were reorganized, I would be unhappy; I like things the way they are.					
7. The opportunity for a career change would frighten me.					
8. When I first hear of a change, I start to think about how bad it will be.					
9. Changes occur too often for me.					
10. New and different work assignments upset me; I try to avoid them.					

Exercise continues on following page 🔷🔷🔷

Scoring

For Questions 1 through 5, give yourself 2 points for every SA and 1 for every A.
_____

SUBTRACT 1 point for every D and 2 for every SD. _____

1 through 5 score = _____

For Questions 6 through 10, give yourself 2 points for every SD and 1 for every D.
_____

SUBTRACT 1 point for every A and 2 for every SA. _____

6 through 10 score = _____

1 through 5 score _____ + 6 through 10 score = _____

If your score is 20 to 13, you cope and adapt to change very well.

If your score is 12 to 4, you cope and adapt to change fairly well.

If your score is 4 to −4, you are ambivalent toward change.

If your score is −5 to −12, you are hesitant to change and adapt slowly.

If your score is −13 to −20, you are reluctant to change and resist adapting to it.

End of exercise. Text continues on following page.

There is almost always something positive in each change. Accepting and coping with change would be far easier if people would look for the good, rather than the bad, in each change. For example, assume that your current work shift has begun at 7:00 am, but now you will have to begin work at 3:30 pm for 1 week out of every 4. What good can be found in this situation? Well, look at it this way—for that 1 week, you will be able to sleep late, avoid rush hour, work with a different clientele, and meet new coworkers. Also, the afternoon shift is typically less noisy, more relaxed (maybe because there are fewer managers around), and sometimes less hectic. Looking for the good in a change can turn what appeared to be a burden into a benefit.

On those rare occasions when you can't find the good right away, it may help to remember that at least the change will break the boredom of doing things the same old way as before. Besides, looking for the positive aspects tends not to excite your systems. Rather than increase your blood pressure fighting change, look for ways in which you will benefit.

Participating in change is not as simple as accepting change, but it may be the most effective way of coping with it.[30] Taking part in the decision-making process for a change or participating in the planning for a change increases cooperation. It is difficult to resist change that you were part of bringing about. It may be that participation is only possible with behavioral managers; however, when any manager asks for managee involvement in a change, it is wise to consider becoming involved. For example, if a manager says that new work assignments are needed and that you will have input into the new assignments, it behooves you to participate.

Learning about a change is a good way to cope with it when participation is not possible. In the process of learning about a change, you will become familiar with it.[31] Often the more familiar you are with a change, the less you will fear it because it will no longer be unknown.[32] Learning about change will also enable you to look for the positive aspects in the change, allowing you to further accept and cope with it. When new procedures are implemented in your area, learning about them may speed your acceptance of them.

Utilization involves using or implementing the change.[33] Utilization can be especially effective with new procedures or equipment.[34] Using a new piece of equipment enables you to cope with it because in using the equipment, you will have to learn about it. Learning about a change and using it will reduce fear of the unknown. Utilization will also provide opportunities for you to find the positive aspects about a change.

Support and assistance involves advocating and sponsoring change and helping others cope with and accept it.[35] Backing a change and educating others about the change requires that you accept it, participate in it, learn about it, and use it. The combination of these activities further increases and all but guarantees your coping with the change. When a new computer system is installed, you could learn about it, discover its advantages, and teach others how to use it as a means of coping with the system yourself.

The final strategy can be used when you have tried the others and discovered that you cannot completely cope with the change as is. *Negotiation* involves discussing the possibility of altering the change to enable someone to cope and comply with it.[36] Typically, the substance of the change remains, whereas the more flexible parts are adjusted. For example, if the department's new forms help the billing department but take the diagnostic and therapeutic areas so long to complete that patient care and efficiency suffer, you should mention this problem to your manager. Point out, in logical and nonthreatening language, that the new forms are having an unforeseen effect on patient care and staff productivity. You may still have to learn to use new forms, but you may be able to negotiate an agreement about new ones that do not detract from operations.

In addition to looking for the beneficial aspects of changes, it may help to understand exactly why the change is being undertaken and what it is supposed to accomplish. In this, you should not consult with your peers. Too often they have no real knowledge so they offer up their best guesses, and this is how rumors get started and communications get misinterpreted. It is best to go to the source. Ask the manager—in a way that does not challenge or threaten—to explain the goals of the change. Possibly explain that if you understood the objective better, you would be better able to implement it. Once you understand what management is trying to accomplish, you should be better able to adjust, accept, and look for the advantages in the new situation. This will make you a better employee and will make your life that much easier and less stressful.

Summary

Change is constantly happening and at an ever-increasing pace. This is true of the health professions more than many other fields. The options are to adapt to it, fight it, or be overcome by it. Being overrun by change is not a viable option for most people who wish to remain active and productive in their chosen professions. Fighting change often serves no useful purpose and often takes its toll only on the managee. For the professional employee in a health-care profession, the only real choice is often to adjust to the change. To do so, you should strive to understand the reason behind the change, look for advantages in the new conditions, select and implement a coping strategy, and accept and implement change to the best advantage for your employer and the least distress for yourself.

REFERENCES

1. Burke, J: The Day the Universe Changed. Little, Brown & Company, Boston, 1985, p 14.
2. Mariotti, J: Troubled by resistance to change? Don't fight it. First, try to understand it. Industry Week. October 7, 1996, pp 30–31.
3. Recardo, R: Process re-engineering in a finance division. Journal for Quality and Participation, June 1994, pp 70–73.
4. Mariotti, pp 30–31.
5. Aldag, RJ, and Stearns, TM: Management, ed 2. Southwestern Publishing, Cincinnati, 1991, p 375.
6. Ibid, p 313.
7. Clark, J, and Kounce, R: Engaging organizational survivors. Train Dev J, August 1995, pp 22–31.
8. Nelson, D, and Quick, J: Organizational Behavior. West, St. Paul, 1994, p 555.
9. Bateman, TS, and Zeithaml, CP: Management: Function and Strategy, ed 2. Irwin, Homewood, Ill., 1993, p 633.
10. Daft, R: Management, ed 5. Dryden, Fort Worth, 2000, p 385.
11. Aldag and Stearns, p 716.
12. Nelson and Quick, p 556.
13. Zimmerman, J: The principle of managing change. HR Focus, February 1995, pp 15–17.
14. Certo, SC: Principle of Modern Management, ed 4. Allyn and Bacon, Boston, 1999, p 299.
15. Nelson and Quick, p 556.
16. Drafke, M, and Kossen, S: The Human Side of Organizations, ed 7. Addison-Wesley Publishing Co, Reading, Mass., 1998, p 347.
17. Herzberg, F: Work and the Nature of Man. World Publishing, Cleveland, 1966.
18. Daft p 372.
19. Nelson and Quick, p 557.
20. Bateman and Zeithaml, p 633.
21. Griffin, RW: Management, ed 6. Houghton Mifflin, Boston, 1999, p 180.
22. Collins, EGC, and Devanna, MA: The Portable MBA. John Wiley & Sons, New York, 1990, p 41.
23. Bateman and Zeithaml, p 637.
24. Nelson and Quick, p 557.
25. Aldag and Stearns, p 718.
26. Certo, p 299.
27. Bateman and Zeithaml, p 627.
28. Collins and Devanna, p 41.
29. Chapman, EN: Supervisor's Survival Kit, ed 6. Macmillan, New York, 1993, p 214.
30. Griffin, p 315.
31. Bateman, and Zeithaml, p 636.
32. Ivancevich, JM, et al: Management: Quality and Competitiveness, ed 2. Irwin, Chicago, 1997, pp 484–490.
33. Mariotti, pp 30–31.
34. Bateman and Zeithaml, p 636.
35. Higgins, JM: The Management Challenge. Macmillan, New York, 1991, p 413.
36. Bateman and Zeithaml, p 636.

11 • Job Satisfaction

Objectives

On completion of this chapter, the reader will be able to:

- ☐ List and define the intrinsic, extrinsic, and personal elements of job satisfaction.
- ☐ Explain the effects that intrinsic, extrinsic, and personal factors have on job satisfaction.
- ☐ List, define, and describe the facets of job satisfaction.
- ☐ Identify working environment characteristics that affect job satisfaction.
- ☐ Describe management's view of the importance of job satisfaction.
- ☐ Summarize the implications of job satisfaction and its complexity.

This chapter is designed to help you identify the factors that affect job satisfaction. This knowledge will allow you to thoroughly examine your job, identify the job satisfaction factors that affect you, and differentiate between the ones that bring satisfaction or dissatisfaction. Once the dissatisfiers have been identified, you may then decide whether they are significant enough for you to take action on them and to decide what kind of action is warranted.

From looking at the chapter outline, you can see that job satisfaction is no longer a simple subject. It was considered so at one time. In the past a job was considered satisfying when the job characteristics met the individual's needs. This single criterion model has since given way to the multidimensional view of today. However, with today's greater understanding of job satisfaction has come a much more complex system. This difference between the past and the present can be readily illustrated with two seemingly simple questions. First ask yourself, "Do I like my job?" The answer will be yes or no. Now ask yourself, "Why?" The old view is like asking if you like your job—"yes" or "no." It is far more difficult to answer the second question completely. Without the material in this chapter, many people might not be able to answer it at all.

Because job satisfaction is somewhat related to motivation, knowledge of that topic is an important prerequisite. Most of this knowledge comes from understanding Maslow's Hierarchy of Needs and Herzberg's theory of hygiene and motivator factors.

Intrinsic Factors of Job Satisfaction

The intrinsic factors of job satisfaction are those most clearly related to the work itself, and these factors are the most difficult to separate from the job. Consequently they are the most difficult to change while continuing to perform the same job.

THE WORK ITSELF

The discussion of job satisfaction both begins and ends with the work itself. To begin with, you must like the work to have any hope at satisfaction. It is difficult to see how someone can be satisfied with work he or she does not like. However, sometimes people say they don't like their jobs and mean that they do not like some *aspect* of the job or that they do not like their *current* job. They still like the profession; they just don't like the way they are practicing it. The ability to make this distinction is one of the primary reasons for including this chapter. Being unable to analyze the job situation and identify the *factor* or *factors* underlying the dissatisfaction will cause some people to leave a profession rather than seek a change in their current job or a different job where those factors are different. Therefore, the steps to take when dissatisfaction is felt are:

1. Analyze the factors presented here.
2. Identify the source of the dissatisfaction.
3. Determine if the factor can be altered and how it can be altered.
4. Act to change the situation.

Beyond the general nature of the work, the following factors have been identified as affecting job satisfaction at the intrinsic level.

VARIETY

Variety refers to the number of skills required to perform a job and the depth of knowledge that must be brought to bear to perform these tasks.[1] Variety is the opposite of job specialization. The effect of job variety is as one would expect—in general, jobs with less variety are less satisfying.[2] In health professions, one can find variations in job variety, even though each profession is relatively well-defined, and practitioners are usually prepared for the whole job. Being prepared for a whole job and only practicing part of it can be a problem for many health professionals in that they are not fully using the skills and knowledge they have acquired. The reasons some people do not use all of their training varies. For example, radiographers are taught to perform all radiographic procedures but may find 30 percent or more of their workload consists of simple, routine chest exams. Or respiratory therapists may feel too intimidated by physicians to give them the full benefit of their knowledge.[3] A solution is to carefully consider the scope of practice required by each position. If skill variety is of high importance to you, give it more weight in considering a job.

AUTONOMY

Autonomy is the degree of freedom people have to control their work.[4] Some health professions are inherently less autonomous than others. Protocols, procedures, and routines are common, with few deviations desired or permitted. However, other forms of autonomy can be used. Health professionals can be given the autonomy to set work hours and their own pace, divide the workload, and so on.[5] Research has shown that as autonomy increases, satisfaction increases. In the studies there were individual variations, however. People with higher-order needs (higher on Maslow's hierarchy) had a stronger desire for autonomy than those with lower-order needs.[6]

GOAL SETTING

Allowing people to *set their own goals* and establish their own criteria for success is not only a motivational technique, it may also increase job satisfaction.[7] On the other hand, it may motivate but not affect job satisfaction.[8] What has been found is that explicit goals are better than ambiguous ones.

RECOGNITION

Receiving *recognition* is frequently mentioned by workers as being a source of satisfaction when it is present and a source of dissatisfaction when it is not.[9] To be effective, the feedback must be accurate (praise for a job well done but also correct when a mistake has been made—correct by identifying who made the mistake and the degree of severity involved)—it must be timely (occurring soon after the incident), and it must happen often (not just at the annual review).[10] When considering prospective employers, ask current employees whether recognition of this type occurs at their workplace.

Other kinds of recognition are more evident because that is their purpose. Awards of the "employee of the month" kind derive almost all of their benefit from the fact that the recognition is visible to others.

Extrinsic Factors of Job Satisfaction

The extrinsic factors of job satisfaction are related to the work or the working environment, but they are either easier to separate from the work or to change than are the intrinsic factors. The extrinsic factors are discussed here according to the control a managee has over them. For example, you can exert more control over how well you do your job (the success factor) than you can over the external opportunities available to someone in your field.

SUCCESS

There is a question about whether *success* on the job causes satisfaction or being satisfied with the job causes success.[11] The distinction may not be as important as the converse situation. People who are unsuccessful at a task are also dissatisfied. The conclusion is that if your work and job satisfaction could use improvement, the place to start may be with your job performance. Do a better job to be more satisfied.

WORK ROLE

Two factors related to your *role at work* can lead to dissatisfaction. One is knowing what your role is. People who are unsure about their position in the formal or informal organizations have higher degrees of role ambiguity than those who know what is expected of them. Higher role ambiguity can lead to higher dissatisfaction.[12]

The other factor is *role conflict*. Role conflict exists when there are discrepancies between one person and another or between one of your roles and another.[13] Increased role conflict produces increased dissatisfaction. The health professions are particularly vulnerable to role conflict problems. The numerous examples of violations of the management law of unity of command are a prime example. The unity of command principle states that each managee should have only one manager. Yet many health professions report to or are accountable to a technical department head (a similar health professional) and a physician. Other factors in the health professions can induce role conflict also. For example, consider the conflict between a manager who instructs you to reduce the use of supplies to save money and the patient's need for those supplies. Or the instructions of a physician that appear to contradict your own training. A code of ethics, professional scope of practice, or accepted standards of behavior may help resolve these situations, but the conflict can still take its toll.

OPPORTUNITIES

Opportunities refers to two factors—long-term opportunities and outside opportunities.[14] If people do not perceive the presence of their *long-term opportunities*, their job satisfaction will decrease. The word *perceive* is very important here. The opportunities they want may be present, but if the employees are not aware of them or if they do not feel that they have a fair chance at them, then they will be less satisfied.

The presence of *outside opportunities* can affect satisfaction in two ways and can also be linked to long-term opportunities. First, the presence of other job options can actually decrease satisfaction with a person's current position: that is, "The grass is always greener on the other side" type of thinking. However, to feel this way, the person must consider these other opportunities to be good. If the conditions of these other jobs are known to be worse (all are part-time when someone wants and needs full-time), the outside opportunities may actually increase satisfaction with a current job.

If a current position does not seem to hold long-term promise, whereas outside opportunities do, satisfaction decreases. However, if a current job does have long-term possibilities and outside opportunities do not or are not present, satisfaction with the present job can increase.

 Building Comprehension Exercise begins on following page

BUILDING COMPREHENSION EXERCISE 11–1

Identifying Intrinsic Factors of Job Satisfaction

Which of these intrinsic factors of job satisfaction are present in your chosen health profession? List examples of each and evaluate how each affects your job satisfaction. Does the presence or absence of the factor contribute a large amount to your job satisfaction (LAJS), does it contribute somewhat to your job satisfaction (SJS), does it not affect your satisfaction (DNA), does it contribute somewhat to dissatisfaction with the job (SD), or does it contribute a large amount to dissatisfaction (LAD)?

	Present	*LAJS*	*SJS*	*DNA*	*SD*	*LAD*	*Example*
Variety	Yes No						
Autonomy	Yes No						
Goal Setting	Yes No						
Recognition	Yes No						

End of exercise. Text continues on following page.

SECURITY

Job security—the level of assurance that one will continue to be employed—is a classic example of Herzberg's hygiene factors.[15] Its importance is increased by its absence. When you have job security, you may not notice it or you may notice it only when examples of low job security are encountered. When you have little job security, you find it is a constant stressor, especially because our society puts great importance on having a job. Job security can be influenced by internal and external factors. Internal factors relate to the employer and manager. Some employers strive to offer job security. Sometimes, though, a particular employer's or manager's attitude may decrease job security because the company or manager constantly reminds managees of the impermanent nature of their jobs. Poor financial condition on the part of the employer is another internal threat to job security.

External factors influencing job security include the economic and political-legal environments. A recession may force cutbacks in employment, although this is not usually a large problem in the health fields. People get sick whether the economy is good or not. The political-legal environment can affect job security in its ability to alter supply and demand. If licensing and credentialing requirements were eliminated, the supply of potential employees would increase. There would be a threat that current workers could be replaced by lower-paid and less-trained new workers. The reverse is also true: Increasing licensing requirements adds to job security.

In any event, there is no question that low job security is related to low job satisfaction.

WORK GROUPS

Maslow, Herzberg, and many others[16] point out the importance that *work groups* and coworkers have on job satisfaction. For many, work may provide more social interactions than nonwork situations. Coinciding with the importance of work relationships is the complexity of trying to understand them. What is understood is that when people's quantity and quality of work group interactions are less than what they desire, their job satisfaction is reduced.

Quantity and quality of interactions are the two main factors connecting work groups and job satisfaction. *Quantity* refers to the number of interactions and is related to the job and working conditions. Sometimes a particular job is performed in relative isolation because of the nature of the work. Such isolation could be physical or mental. *Physical isolation* means there are simply no other workers around; for instance this occurs when you are working in satellite or mobile situations or in an x-ray darkroom. *Mental isolation* means that although many other people are around, the concentration level the job requires is so high that it's almost the same as working alone. Some medical laboratory positions (for instance, a cytotechnologist) are like this. When it is the nature of the work that creates isolation, you should make sure you are available to socialize with other coworkers. In addition, joining your professional society may help.

The matter of the *quality* of work group contacts is much more subjective. It is also very powerful. People have remained at jobs they otherwise would have left because they like the people, patients, or clients. Others have left (or been driven from) jobs that were perfectly acceptable because of the people they came into contact with. Although it is not the purpose of this book to completely discuss group dynamics, there are things you can do that may help in working with others.

Some of the things that can be done to smooth working relationships appear, at first glance, to be simple and obvious. However, it is absolutely amazing how many people ignore them in real life. The first thing is also one that typically earns the most respect from peers: job knowledge. Know your job and know it well. But that is only half of the story. You must also *perform* your job. There are people who are very good at what they do; they are just too lazy to do much of it. If you want to get along with your colleagues at work, know your job and do your job. Next you might expect a long list of do's and don'ts, and it is certainly possible to compile one. It is almost certain that the list will (1) never be learned or (2) never be remembered. Fortunately, it is also possible to cover the same material with one rule. However, this rule is not new and is probably something everyone learned before: Do unto others as you would have them do unto you. In other words, treat people the way you want to be treated. This applies to coworkers, bosses, patients, and clients. Be forewarned that applying this rule is not easy. Certainly there will be people who will not reciprocate, but your applying the rule is professional and probably has the greatest chance of yielding positive results.

MANAGEMENT

The quality of supervision is another of Herzberg's hygiene factors. A "good" supervisor may not make you like a "bad" job, but a "bad" supervisor can make you dislike a "good" job.[17] It may appear that this is one of the factors that you have little or no control over, and to a certain degree that is true.

Many times, however, managers do not manage because of the way they are; they manage the way a managee makes them. Some people's work habits are not very good. This may cause a manager who is otherwise behavioral to manage that person in an authoritarian way. Others who are performing their jobs in an orderly, proficient manner may receive entirely different treatment from this exact same manager. Let me make it perfectly clear what I am, and am *not,* advocating here. I am *not* advocating ingratiation with a manager to receive the desired treatment. I am saying that you can influence some managers so you are treated the way you wish to be by doing your job well and by treating them with respect and professionalism.

THE ORGANIZATION

In addition to individual managers and supervisors who use an authoritarian or a behavioral style of management, entire *organizations* can also use these styles. Authoritarian organizations are typically called "bureaucratic." They do not take the feelings of individuals into account, nor do they recognize or consider the informal organization. Unfortunately, the majority of organizations are bureaucratic.[18] Job satisfaction is generally higher in nonbureaucratic organizations.[19]

SCHEDULING

Some companies have found that altering *scheduling* helps people feel more satisfied.[20] The two main forms have been to extend weekends and to give workers some control over their hours. Weekends are extended by compressing the workweek. Typically, four 10-hour days are worked, rather than five 8-hour days. There are even some instances where two 16-hour shifts on Saturday and Sunday are worked, for which 40 hours are paid. In terms of increasing worker control, these scheduling arrangements may include (1) freely allowing workers to exchange days worked, (2) allowing workers to schedule themselves for the days they wish, or (3) permitting people to begin work within a certain time—let's say, between 7:30 AM and 9:00 AM—and finish 8 hours later. The effects on job satisfaction of compressed workweeks and flextime are similar to those of Herzberg's hygiene factors. Their use may not increase satisfaction (or increase it slightly), but scheduling that increases stress and demands on workers may increase dissatisfaction. It can also be difficult to offer these options to some health-care professions because some departments must be staffed 24 hours a day and others have constant patient demands. These patient demands can range from patients' needing treatment at specific times to patients' needing to schedule appointments. One can't tell a patient he or she will be seen sometime between 7:30 AM and 9:30 AM, because his appointment depends on when a worker feels like coming in.

TIME

The amount of *time* someone has spent in a position affects job satisfaction, but the time element is a unreliable element in predicting exactly how satisfaction will be affected.[21] For some, job satisfaction increases over time because they perform at a higher level. For others, satisfaction decreases because over time work has become boring or they realize that their aspirations are not being met. When satisfaction decreases because of the amount of time spent on the job, the solution some people choose is to leave that position. This may mean applying for a promotion, making a lateral move to another profession, moving to another employer, or leaving the health-care field altogether. Most employers will understand an employee who requests some job changes; however, employers may question numerous changes, especially if they occur after working only a few months in a particular position.

MONEY

When most people are asked, "Why do you work?", the response is almost assuredly, "For money." Certainly *money* is a major reason to work, and a certain amount of it is satisfying. For example, money satisfies physiologic and status needs on Maslow's hierarchy. However, money is only part of the picture. As we have seen, money may be an important reason to work, but it is certainly not the *only* reason for many people.[22] Although money does provide a certain amount of satisfaction, does more money mean people will be more satisfied? Many people would say "yes" and promptly ask for more. However, money may not be the right motivator for action in every situation.

People sometimes ask for more money when a lack of money is not the real problem. An examination of why this request occurs may help you avoid the problem. First of all, people ask for more money because it is viewed by most people as suitable compensation for a lack of other satisfiers. Certain jobs warrant more pay because they are so boring that people won't do them. Money compensates these people for not having an interesting job. However, there can come a point when the factor for which money is supposed to compensate becomes unbearable. Here, people frequently ask for more money. Sometimes, the palliative effect is rather short lived. In the short term, the increased money alleviates a feeling that a job is unbearable, but the worker eventually needs more money. This is why Herzberg calls money a hygiene factor. He calls the situation of constantly needing higher and higher rewards "jumping for the jelly beans." To get a person to work, he or she must be given a reward (a jelly bean). For more work, he or she needs more reward (more jelly beans). But then performance will drop back to its former level, even though the reward is greater, so more reward must be given. Because the root of the problem— the unbearableness of the factor being compensated for—is never addressed, money can never satisfy it.

Other reasons people ask for increases in money include tangibility, objectivity, foolishness, and symbolism. *Tangibility* refers to the fact that money is a concrete reward. It is palpable and there for all to see. The psychological rewards of work are also important, but they are intangible. It can be difficult or impossible for others to see that work, for you, has become more interesting or more enjoyable.

The fact that money has more *objectivity* than many other rewards is another reason why people ask for it. It is easily measured, and you always know when you are getting more or less of it. It is more difficult to find work that is more exciting than your current job. Job excitement is hard to measure. You may be the only one to know what is more exciting and what is not, and sometimes that can be difficult to put into words. It is not easy to give people subjective rewards like this.

For these reasons and others (such as money being a time-honored, acceptable reward), some people feel a little *foolish* asking for other types of reimbursement. Rather than ask for a job with less stress or one with more creativity or fewer hassles, some ask for only more money. If this happens to you, don't be too surprised if the effects of increased pay last only a short time.

Finally, money is *symbolic*. It represents status to coworkers and society in general. It is also important to some people as a reinforcement of their achievements and of their self-worth. It is a way of keeping score with how you are doing.

Money does not solve all problems. It is here where an understanding of money can be most helpful. As Herzberg and others believe, money is only a temporary satisfier or it is a dissatisfier. In many cases, people use money to treat a *symptom,* instead of a *problem*. To avoid this, you should al-ways ask yourself, "What is the *real* problem? Will more money correct that problem?" There are cases when, for whatever reasons, people need more money. In these cases, they must then decide whether or not they can meet their needs in their current position and their current profession. At other times, the problem is not related to money. In these situations, money will not change the situation and may provide only temporary relief. In the long run it will be better in these situations to find out what the real problem is and what will solve this problem, and then seek it out. Maybe you need more responsibility. Maybe you need less. Maybe you need a greater or lesser challenge. Or it is quite possible that the problem is not related to your job. It may be a personal problem that is affecting your work, but you may not realize it until you analyze the situation. Therefore, to maximize satisfaction, you need to know what satisfiers exist, and in what way they can satisfy you. Then you must obtain the satisfiers with the minimum amount of compromise and substitution.

Personal Factors of Job Satisfaction

Not all job satisfaction comes from the job. There are a number of personal factors that impact how a person feels about his or her job. They are essentially beyond the control of managers, and some are beyond the "control" of the managee. Even though you may not be able to control the factor, an understanding of what the factor is and knowing that it affects you may enable you to mentally remove it as a source of dissatisfaction.

PERSONAL COMMITMENT

For allied health professionals, *personal commitment* can be one of the major personal factors affecting job satisfaction. Personal commitment means that someone has researched various jobs, carefully selected a career, and invested time or money or both to learn the job.[23] The greater these efforts are and the more friends and family know about these efforts, the higher is the personal commitment, which can mean greater satisfaction. It may also mean that the person is less likely to admit that the profession is not satisfying. To do so would be to admit a mistake—a mistake that it appears should not have been made, given the effort invested in making the selection. Unfortunately, instead of admitting that the job is not satisfying and finding one that is, some people stay on and remain dissatisfied.

 Building Comprehension Exercise begins on following page

BUILDING COMPREHENSION EXERCISE 11–2

Identifying Extrinsic Factors of Job Satisfaction

Which of these intrinsic factors of job satisfaction are present in your chosen health profession? List examples of each and evaluate how each affects your job satisfaction. Does the presence or absence of the factor contribute a large amount to your job satisfaction (LAJS), does it contribute somewhat to your job satisfaction (SJS), does it not affect your satisfaction (DNA), does it contribute somewhat to dissatisfaction with the job (SD), or does it contribute a large amount to dissatisfaction (LAD)?

	Present	LAJS	SJS	DNA	SD	LAD	Example
Success	Yes No						
Work Role	Yes No						
Opportunities	Yes No						
Security	Yes No						
Work Groups	Yes No						

Exercise continues on following page ❧❧❧

	Present	*LAJS*	*SJS*	*DNA*	*SD*	*LAD*	*Example*
Management	Yes No						
The Organization	Yes No						
Scheduling	Yes No						
Time	Yes No						
Money	Yes No						

End of exercise. Text continues on following page.

JOB EXPECTATIONS

Job expectations are those outcomes managees believe they will receive from a job.[24] If they have high expectations and the reality of the job does not measure up, they will be disappointed. On the other hand, if expectations are low and the outcomes are low, they may have less dissatisfaction.

Unfulfilled job expectations can also occur when people expect their jobs to fulfill all of their needs. Our society puts a high value on employment, so high that some may believe that work should fulfill all their needs. In actuality, many positions will not be able to do that. This can be true of the health professions because of their typically short promotion ladder. In fact, for many health professions the only movement available is to change careers—laterally to another health field, to management, or to education. If health-care practitioners have a need for status or increased responsibility, they may feel stifled by the existing organization structure. This is another time when knowledge of Maslow's hierarchy can be useful. It can tell you when you are at the point where status may fulfill your needs. It does not say that those needs must be fulfilled from your job. Actually, there are many roles outside work through which people may find status and recognition, namely, volunteer and professional organizations. This fulfillment helps explain why so many people work so hard for no "pay."

TASK IMPORTANCE

Task importance is the degree of importance the job has in a person's life.[25] People who are more involved with their work often have more job satisfaction.[26] However, it is possible to have too much involvement with a job. Sometimes a "workaholic's" personal life suffers from this overcommitment.[27]

EFFORT COMPARED TO REWARDS

People *compare the effort* they put into a job to *the rewards* they receive when determining job satisfaction.[28] This works much like the equity theory of motivation. If people feel they are putting more into their work than they are getting out, they will not feel satisfied. If they believe that their effort-reward ratio is less than their coworkers' effort-reward ratio, they will not feel satisfied. The reward aspect often refers to more than just monetary compensation. It refers to all the rewards—perceived and actual. This would include recognition, respect, and so on.

COWORKERS

Coworkers can influence job satisfaction through means other than effort-reward comparisons. Whatever coworkers frequently discuss among themselves will take on more importance than topics not discussed.[29] If your coworkers talk about what great work schedules they have, you will see schedules as an important topic; if your schedule is not so great, you will be more dissatisfied than if the topic had not been discussed. This influence also happens when coworkers talk about how bad a work situation is or how a particular profession is not very good. Others will be influenced by this and often agree (of course, if a situation is so bad, why do the people complaining about it stay?).

COMPARISONS TO OTHERS

People view their jobs in relation to coworkers and also in relation to friends and relatives. If you feel that your friends and relatives have better jobs than you, you will have more dissatisfaction than if you believe you are all equal.[30]

OTHER PEOPLE'S OPINIONS

The way you feel about your job may also be influenced by the way others view it. If others, especially those you regarded highly, feel that you have a good job or feel that your job should provide you with satisfaction, you will be more satisfied than if they did not think this way.[31] This applies to the way society views entire professions. Fortunately, most people feel that being in a health profession is a worthy job and that helping people should be satisfying and rewarding.

SELF-ESTEEM AND SELF-CONFIDENCE

Your view of yourself, that is, your self-worth and self-confidence, can affect your job satisfaction. If you are confident and have a positive outlook on yourself and life in general, it is more likely that you will be satisfied with the work you do.[32]

AGE

In general, job satisfaction increases as people get older.[33] It is felt that this is because of experience and a more realistic view of work. Younger workers have few work experiences with which to compare

 Building Comprehension Exercise begins on following page

BUILDING COMPREHENSION EXERCISE 11–3

Evaluating Personal Factors of Job Satisfaction

Evaluate how each of these personal factors affects your job satisfaction. Does the presence or absence of the factor contribute a large amount to your job satisfaction (LAJS), does it contribute somewhat to your job satisfaction (SJS), does it not affect your satisfaction (DNA), does it contribute somewhat to dissatisfaction with the job (SD), or does it contribute a large amount to dissatisfaction (LAD)? List examples of each.

	LAJS	*SJS*	*DNA*	*SD*	*LAD*	*Example*
Personal Commitment						
Job Expectations						
Task Importance						
Effort Compared to Rewards						
Coworkers						
Comparisons to Others						

Exercise continues on following page ❖ ❖ ❖

	LAJS	SJS	DNA	SD	LAD	Example
Other People's Opinions						
Self-esteem						
Self-confidence						

End of exercise. Text continues on following page.

their current positions. They may substitute the opinions of others, their beliefs of how other people's jobs are, and their own idealistic notions of what work should be. The greater experiences of the older worker help that person realize what a job is—and is not. This knowledge then leads to a more realistic view of life and the place of work in that life. If a young worker has an idealistic view that is not matched by the job, he or she will be less satisfied than an older worker who had the same job experience but a more realistic view of what to expect. It is not so much the amount of job satisfaction a position yields (if that could even be measured), but the *difference* between what we expect and what we get. The greater the difference, the less satisfied we are.

Management's View

Managers have a number of views on job satisfaction mainly centering on the relationship between job satisfaction and performance. The reason there are differing opinions is that the research is not conclusive. Some find that if workers have high performance, they are more satisfied.[34] Others find that workers with high job satisfaction perform better.[35] The truth may be entirely different. Possibly the only important fact is that the two are related, so managers should be as concerned about job satisfaction as the managees are.

One correlation with job satisfaction that is not in dispute is the relationship between satisfaction and absenteeism and turnover.[36] Both are costly to organizations, and both increase as satisfaction decreases. One might think that management would be more concerned with job satisfaction in areas with high turnover and absenteeism. However, sometimes management attributes high turnover or absenteeism to the basic nature of the job. It is assumed to be a cost of doing business, and instead of having more concern for it and job satisfaction, there is actually less.

Summary

Two dozen factors that influence job satisfaction have been introduced and discussed. Why? Well, some of the things that separate modern workers from those of the past are that they expect more from work and they have more choices before them. Still, many people appear less than satisfied with their work, but they don't seem to know what to do about it. This, then, is the purpose of

this chapter. To provide the means by which someone can analyze his or her situation and do something about it. Maybe there is a problem with an internal factor, a factor so basic that a person would have to leave the profession to avoid it. For example, some people, during the first weeks of an educational program, discover that they really don't like working with sick people. Sometimes it takes longer. If this is true, a change to a nonpatient, or nonclient, medical field is necessary, or perhaps even a change to a nonmedical job. Or the problem may be with the current working conditions and not the profession. It would be better for these people to know this and change their work shifts, departments, or jobs than to leave a profession that could have satisfied them. Finally, the problem may be with the person, and this is just as important for a person to know, although it is sometimes harder for them to admit.

REFERENCES

1. Lam, Simon, SK: Quality managment and job satisfaction. International Journal of Quality and Reliability Management, April 1995, pp 72–79.
2. Gruneberg, MM: Understanding Job Satisfaction. John Wiley & Sons, New York, 1979, p 43.
3. Smith, R: A paradigm for satisfaction. The Journal for Respiratory Care Practitioners, June/July 1992, pp 62–69.
4. Dilworth, J: Operations Management, ed. 3. Dryden, Fort Worth, 2000, p 306.
5. Smith, p 68.
6. Gruneberg, p 45.
7. Lowenberg, G, and Conrad, K: Current Perspectives in Industrial/Organizational Psychology. Allyn and Bacon, Needham Heights, Mass., 1998, pp 350–52.
8. Gruneberg, p 35.
9. Leslie, AW, and Redmon, WK: The effects of feedback and goal setting on the productivity and satisfaction of university admissions staff. Journal of Organizational Behavior Management, Winter, 1998, pp 45–65.
10. Lowenberg and Conrad, pp 189–90.
11. Gruneberg, p 34.
12. Shelledy, DC, et al: Analysis of job satisfaction, burnout, and intent of respiratory care practitioners to leave the field of the job. Respir Care 37(1):46–60, 1992.
13. Nelson, D, and Quick, J: Organizational Behavior. West, St. Paul, 1994, pp 396–98.
14. Lowenberg and Conrad, p 374.
15. French, W: Human Resources Management, ed 2. Houghton Mifflin, Boston, 1990, p 126.
16. Gruneberg, p 64.
17. Nelson, and Quick, p 149.
18. Argyris, C: Personality and organization theory revisited. Adm Sci Q 18:141–67, 1973.
19. Gruneberg, MM, p 84.
20. Bergen, K: Timely exercise: Compact schedules help workers stretch. Chicago Tribune, March 2, 1997; sect 5:1, 6.
21. Gruneberg, MM, p 93.
22. Gini, AR, and Sullivan, TJ: It Comes with the Territory: An Inquiry Concerning Work and the Person. Random House, New York, 1989, p 17.
23. Strauss, G, and Sayles, LR: Behavioral Strategies for Managers. Prentice-Hall, Englewood Cliffs, NJ, 1980, p 17.

24. Ibid, p 17.
25. Dilworth, p 306.
26. Gruneberg, p 35.
27. Aldag, RJ, and Stearns, TM: Management, ed 2. Southwestern Publishing, Cincinnati, 1991, p 393.
28. Lowenberg and Conrad, pp 374–78.
29. Strauss and Sayles, p 17.
30. Strauss and Sayles, p 17.
31. Strauss and Sayles, p 17.
32. Strauss and Sayles, p 17.
33. Lowenberg and Conrad, pp 371–72.
34. Scott, WR: Organizations: Rational, Natural and Open Systems, ed 2. Prentice-Hall, Englewood Cliffs, NJ, 1987, p 61.
35. Vecchio, R: Organizational Behavior, ed. 3. Dryden, Fort Worth, 1995, p 134.
36. Scott, p 61.

12 · Introduction to Stress

Objectives

On completion of this chapter, the reader will be able to:

- ☐ Define stress.
- ☐ Differentiate eustress and distress.
- ☐ Describe responses to stress.
- ☐ Describe reactions to stress.
- ☐ Identify and define work-related stressors.
- ☐ Identify, define, and explain work-related stress reactions.
- ☐ Describe general stress management techniques for the working environment.
- ☐ Describe general stress management techniques for outside the working environment.

People need stress to survive.[1] An absence of stress, or sensory deprivation, causes death. However, too much of the wrong kind of stress is also bad. This chapter will introduce stress terms, general concepts, and stress as it relates to the working environment. Responses, reactions, and methods of coping with stress will also be discussed. The intention here is to alert people to the effects of stress. This chapter will outline, but not detail, methods for coping with stress. The overall goal is to diagram stress and describe strategies that could be employed to manage it after further research or with professional assistance.

Understanding Stress

Much of the research into stress was conducted by Dr. Hans Selye (pronounced Sell-yeä). He produced a large amount of the basic data on stress, types of stress, causes of stress, and reactions to stress. It was his work that demonstrated the physiologic result of too much bad stress. He also described good stress and methods for coping with stress in general.

DEFINITIONS

Dr. Selye defines *stress* as the body's nonspecific response to any demand.[2] In other words, the body has a general reaction to any tension placed on it. Anything that produces a demand is called a *stressor*.[3] Stress that is bad for us, that is unpleasant or disease producing, is called *distress*.[4] Stress that is good, or curative, is termed *eustress* (pronounced you-stress).[5]

The same general activity may produce bad stress or good stress, depending on the specifics of the situation and the individual. For example, being chased is a stressor. If you are being chased by a mugger, it is distress. Repeated occurrences are probably be harmful, even if the mugger never catches you. However, being chased by someone as part of a game or in a recreational sport is a form of eustress. Repeated exposure does not harm you and is actually good for you.

The example just given is also one of *physical stress*. Being chased by a mugger is an example of physical distress, and being chased as part of a game is an example of physical eustress. Most modern people are more often, though not exclusively, exposed to *emotional* (or mental) *distress* and eustress. Although we each have a certain, individual level of adaptation or reaction to stress, our basic responses to it are limited and very primitive.

BASIC RESPONSES

We have two basic responses to stress—fight or flight.[6] The *fight response* is the more severe of the two. The individual prepares to defend himself or herself, elevating the capabilities of some systems and depressing others. Adrenalin output increases, and heart rate, blood pressure, and respirations rise.[7] However, the digestive system is shut down because it is not needed for defense.[8] Blood is diverted from it to the skeletal muscles. The entire organism is now on full alert.[9] This system serves people well when they are faced with physical distress, which was vastly more common in the ancient past than it is today. However, we have yet to develop alternative alert systems for the emotional distress found in the modern world.

The *flight response* prepares us to escape to avoid the stressor, rather than battle against it. It is a lesser response than the fight response and produces less tension. Fewer, and different, hormones are released. Less strenuous nervous stimuli are evident, and the organism is under less pressure.[10]

Individuals have their own levels of tolerance for stress, over which they can exercise some control. Selecting the way in which you respond to distress forms your reaction to stress.

BASIC REACTIONS

There are two basic reactions to stress from which to choose, just as there are two basic responses. Choosing to respond to distress with a fight response is a *catatoxic reaction;* choosing a flight response is a *syntoxic reaction.*[11]

Selecting a catatoxic reaction to distress is, in general, bad. There are times when a fight response is called for, for example, in a life-threatening situation. Most modern distress, however, is emotional or mental. The problem with selecting a catatoxic reaction to emotional distress is that you are trying to use a physical response to a mental threat. In almost all cases, there is no physical outlet for the fight response. The body's battle systems are at a heightened state, but in a modern work situation they have nothing to do. With no release, the hormonal and nervous stimuli are turned inward and work against you.[12] The increase in blood pressure, increase in muscle tension, blood transfer from the alimentary canal to the skeletal muscles, and increases in gastric secretions cause a number of detrimental effects.[13] These include spasms of the gastrointestinal (GI) tract, increased pulse rate, cardiovascular disease, and gastric and duodenal ulcers.[14] Fortunately, there is an alternative.

It is possible to develop syntoxic responses to stress.[15] A syntoxic response means that you do not get aroused, angry, irritated, or upset in the face of emotional or mental distress. You do not allow yourself to have an agitated response to something you cannot change. If the stressor is not one that you can alter, a catatoxic response hurts no one but yourself.

For instance, your boss walks by for the first time today; it happens to be the *only* moment you have had to catch your breath, and he remarks about how nice it must be to have such an easy a job, and then he leaves. A catatoxic reaction would be to get angry, maybe mumble something about the boss, throw a few things around or vent your anger on a coworker or patient. What is accomplished by doing this? Nothing good! The boss is gone and knows nothing of your dislike and disagreement with his remarks. All that has been done is that *your* systems are on alert. *Your* head is throbbing. *Your* GI tract is attacking itself. *Your* patient receives inferior care. All for no purpose and to no avail. On the other hand, a person selecting a syntoxic response might think, "Well, he wasn't around all morning to see what really happened and probably didn't mean anything by what he said." Or maybe, "I can't believe someone that out of touch with his department still has a job here." Or even, "What a jerk! That was totally inappropriate and unprofessional. Certainly no way to keep or motivate employees. Oh well, that's *his* problem." Some may call this rationalization, but that is not important. Whatever you think of is probably okay if it keeps you from having a fight response and gearing up all your systems for nothing.

Now, if you are thinking that developing syntoxic reactions is easier said than done, especially with the pace and pressure of modern life, you are quite right. Dr. Selye, who writes in depth on developing syntoxic reactions, admits that they do not come easily or instantly. He points out that you must make a constant, conscious effort to cultivate them. The process could even take years, but few things that are worthwhile are quickly obtained. The choice is to face a lifetime of angry, self-defeating reactions that can easily lead to pain and disease or to invest some time and effort to develop syntoxic reactions that are almost automatic. Surely the latter seems a much better choice.

It must also be realized that a catatoxic response is inappropriate even for situations you can change. Studies have shown that the best way to accomplish objectives within an organization is to remain calm and use a logical approach.[16] A civilized, rational, syntoxic response produces the best results.

Causes of Stress

The causes of stress are numerous and certainly not limited to the workplace. The emphasis here, however, will be on stress that involves working. Most of the stressors introduced here concern the working environment, but basic coping strategies for work-related stress will include a discussion of support from outside the workplace as well.

WORK-RELATED STRESSORS

The main area to be examined here involves stressors related to working. *Quantitative* and *qualitative demands* refer to work output. *Control* refers to the pace of the work. *Participation* concerns work and social contacts. The *type of shift* that is worked affects stress levels, whereas *work roles* refer to the parts people play at work. *A person's age combined with the amount of time he or she works each week* also contributes to stress. Finally, a combination of a number of factors can produce *chronic stress*.

Quantitative demands can produce distress in four ways that include the amount of work, the time allotted, the repetitiveness of the work, and the amount of attention or concentration required.[17-19] Asking people to produce more work than they are capable of can produce distress. Generally, increased workloads can be managed for a day or a few days. However, if an area is understaffed for an extended period (due to a decrease in workers or an increase in work), the effects of this stress become evident. Typical responses range from workers' being irritable with each other or with patients and clients, to absenteeism and resignation. Likewise, if the time allotted to complete work is decreased, detrimental effects will be seen in the long run. Work that is highly repetitive, where there is little chance for variety or change, produces distress. Jobs requiring high levels of concentration also produce distress and tensions.

Qualitative demands produce distress when the job content is too narrow.[20,21] Narrowness of job content is related to the tolerances of each individual worker. Factors that contribute to a job's being too narrow include a lack of variety in the tasks performed, no opportunities for problem solving or chances to use one's creativity, and few social contacts available through a person's work.

Not being able to *control* the speed of the workplace or the methods for completing work can cause distress.[22] Both of these examples relate to the degree of autonomy workers are given, which will be discussed later in this chapter.

A low level of *participation* can produce distress for those who want to make a contribution.[23] Distress from a lack of participation can be caused by working in isolation and includes being physically separated from others or temporally separated (working the night shift and having few contacts as a result). The effects of this isolation can include

 Building Comprehension Exercise begins on following page

BUILDING COMPREHENSION EXERCISE 12–1

Rating Work-related Stressors

Circle the points that represent the degree to which each factor affects you. Explain how each factor affects you and the reason for your rating.

	Much Greater Than I Am Comfortable with	Greater Than I Am Comfortable with	Just Right	Somewhat Less Than I Am Comfortable with	Much Less Than I Am Comfortable with
Amount of work	4 points	2 points	(0 points)	1 point	3 points

Explain

	Much Greater Than I Am Comfortable with	Greater Than I Am Comfortable with	Just Right	Somewhat Less Than I Am Comfortable with	Much Less Than I Am Comfortable with
Variety of tasks I perform	3 points	1 point	(0 points)	2 points	4 points

Explain

	Much Greater Than I Am Comfortable with	Greater Than I Am Comfortable with	Just Right	Somewhat Less Than I Am Comfortable with	Much Less Than I Am Comfortable with
Repetitiveness of my work	4 points	2 points	0 points	(1 point)	3 points

Explain

	Much Greater Than I Am Comfortable with	Greater Than I Am Comfortable with	Just Right	Somewhat Less Than I Am Comfortable with	Much Less Than I Am Comfortable with
Concentration required for my work	4 points	2 points	(0 points)	1 point	3 points

Explain

	Much Greater Than I Am Comfortable with	Greater Than I Am Comfortable with	Just Right	Somewhat Less Than I Am Comfortable with	Much Less Than I Am Comfortable with
Time allotted for my work	2 points	1 point	(0 points)	3 points	4 points

Explain

Exercise continues on following page ⬡⬡⬡

	Much Greater Than I Am Comfortable with	Greater Than I Am Comfortable with	Just Right	Somewhat Less Than I Am Comfortable with	Much Less Than I Am Comfortable with
Opportunities for problem solving	3 points	1 point	0 points	(2 points)	4 points

Explain

	Much Greater Than I Am Comfortable with	Greater Than I Am Comfortable with	Just Right	Somewhat Less Than I Am Comfortable with	Much Less Than I Am Comfortable with
Chances to use creativity	3 points	1 point	0 points	2 points	(4 points)

Explain

	Much Greater Than I Am Comfortable with	Greater Than I Am Comfortable with	Just Right	Somewhat Less Than I Am Comfortable with	Much Less Than I Am Comfortable with
Social contacts	2 points	1 point	(0 points)	3 points	4 points

Explain

Total the points and check how work-related stressors contribute to your general level of stress.

0–4 points—You perceive almost no distress from these factors.

5–13 points—You perceive a relatively low amount of distress from these factors.

14–24 points—You perceive a moderate amount of distress from these factors.

25–32 points—You perceive a relatively large amount of distress from these factors.

End of exercise. Text continues on following page.

the creation of passive workers and feelings of social helplessness. Not being part of the decision-making process can also produce distress from a feeling of nonparticipation.

The *work shift* that a person is assigned to can cause increased stress in a number of ways.[24] First, if a person's work shift changes, commonly known as *working swing shifts,* the normal, circadian body rhythms can become disrupted. This change upsets the body's internal clock and compounds existing mental, physical, and social problems. It can also cause digestive and sleep disorders. These problems can also be compounded in someone working only the night shift if the adjustment to night work is not made. These conditions have been found to decrease when night work ceases. Studies have also found that absenteeism from night work is similar to that from day work, except for older workers. Older workers' absenteeism increased on the night shifts. Of course, a major social concern of evening and night shift work is that workers are out of synchronization with the majority of the population. Decreased contact with friends and family should be considered if you are contemplating one of these shifts.

Work roles contribute to work stress through role ambiguity and role conflict. Both impact the various parts people play in the formal and informal organizations.

Role ambiguity can be caused by confusion with your role in the formal organization, in the informal organization, or both.[25] Confusion from a formal organization role can come from a lack of information on exactly what that role entails. This may be due to a nonexistent or poorly written job description or from a boss who has not detailed your duties, is vague about your duties, or is constantly changing them. Role ambiguity increases stress in the form of increased tension. Physically, this can cause elevated blood pressure and a higher pulse rate. Mentally, ambiguity manifests itself in decreased job satisfaction and lower self-confidence.

Role conflict can be caused by demands placed on you that contradict one another or that are mutually exclusive. Role conflict can also result from having to perform tasks that you do not want to perform or that you feel are not part of your responsibility. The physical manifestation of role conflict is increased heart rate.[26]

Length of the workweek can contribute to work stress for people younger than age 45 if they work more than 48 hours per week. These people have twice the risk of dying from coronary artery disease as those not working under these conditions.[27]

Both psychological and psychosomatic problems can result from *chronic stressors.*[28] Such long-term frustration from overpromotion, underpromotion, lack of job security, and thwarted ambition can have detrimental effects. *Overpromotion* stress, also known as the "Peter principle," can result when someone is promoted beyond his or her ability. However, *underpromotion* may also cause increased distress. This happens when people are ready, willing, and able to take on additional responsibilities, but are not given them. It is easily understood how lack of job security can produce increased distress and tension, as can having your goals or ambitions blocked.

NON-WORK-RELATED STRESSORS

The stressors just described have all been directly related to job tasks or the job itself. However, job stress may be indirectly related to work, in the form of social supports.

The stress caused by *social support* is commonly distress and is caused by a lack of support.[29] This lack may be from family, friends, or coworkers. Furthermore, it may be active or passive. *Active nonsupport* means that people deride, discount, or belittle your job. *Passive nonsupport* means that backing for you in your job is missing. Active nonsupport means that someone is telling you that they think very little of your job. Passive nonsupport means that no one is saying anything bad about your job, but no one is saying anything good about it either.

It is possible that a lack of social support can be transitory. For instance, sometimes a lack of social support is because of a misunderstanding or a lack of knowledge as to the exact nature of the job. Once the vital role a particular health profession plays in health care in general is explained, friends and family may change their opinions. Or the lack of support may be because coworkers are unsure of your abilities because you are new to the department or new to the position. Once you have proven yourself knowledgeable and capable, they may support you.

Having outlined the basic causes of work stress, it is possible to proceed to the reactions they cause.

Work-related Stress Reactions

Work distress may cause affective, behavioral, or physical reactions. Affective reactions are emotionally based. Behavioral reactions demonstrate themselves in our actions. Physical reactions are manifest through physiologic changes. Work distress may cause reactions in one, two, or all three categories. Also, a person may exhibit one or more of the reactions within a category, or he or she may present with one or more reactions from all categories.

AFFECTIVE REACTIONS

Affective reactions involve emotions, rather than conscious thought. They are subjective, rather than objective.[30] Repression of emotional reactions may lead to illness.[31] It is possible that containing them may lead to depression.[32] However, it is not usually possible, or else it is not usually advisable, to vent hostilities or other emotions in the workplace. Releasing emotions on unsuspecting patients, clients, bosses, or coworkers is counterproductive. It may become necessary, if emotional levels build too high, to find alternative coping or release measures (these are described in the stress management section).

BEHAVIORAL REACTIONS

Behavioral reactions to work stress are quite common and can be divided into four categories: substance abuse, active behaviors, passive behaviors, and other behaviors.[33]

Substance abuse is so problematic that it is currently a national issue receiving much attention. It includes abuse of legal, illegal, and prescription drugs. Although treatment programs are numerous, their effectiveness may be called into question if the cause of the abuse is work-related stress that is not addressed or if the stress-producing conditions are not altered.

Active behaviors generally include some form of escape from the work stressors. A person may engage in a work slowdown in which he or she deliberately reduces the pace. Or an employee may be reluctant to perform certain tasks. The ultimate form of escaping work distress is to resign. Through each of these actions, the person is attempting to reduce distress by avoiding the stressors.

Passive behaviors are not as evident in the quantity of work produced. Instead, the quality of work may decline, and the person may be uninterested in correcting it. Or the person may lack motivation. Instead of maintaining at least a semblance of interest in working, the person may become indifferent. He or she may become apathetic, lethargic, disinterested, or incurious about the job. Instead of escapist, these behaviors are more defeatist, more like surrendering.

Other behaviors that are seen include an increase in accidents, a decrease in participation, and a decrease in productivity. Increased accident rates and a decrease in participation are more closely associated with the passive behaviors. A person less interested in a job is more prone to become careless and thus suffer more accidents. It is also easy to envision someone unconcerned with work being uninterested in participating on the job. Decreases in productivity, on the other hand, may be associated with any of the other behaviors. Substance abuse, active behaviors, and passive behaviors all contribute to lower quantity and quality of work, thereby decreasing productivity.

PHYSICAL REACTIONS

Physical reactions can produce changes in anatomy and physiology. Basic reactions can be divided into those seen in the alimentary canal, the circulatory system, and other systems.

Reactions to distress that are evident in the *alimentary canal* may occur at almost any point. At the proximal end there may be dryness of the mouth and the throat and an increase in the production of gastric digestive juices.[34] This reaction may lead to the formation of gastric or duodenal ulcers.[35] On the other hand, the stomach, small bowel, and colon are all susceptible to stress-induced spasm.[36]

Disturbances of the *circulatory system* from distress vary in severity. Temporary increases in the pulse rate are possible and may have a limited overall effect.[37] Increased blood pressure is also possible and, if chronic, can be quite damaging.[38] Cardiovascular heart disease is also possible and is a major cause of death in the United States.[39]

Other systems that may be affected by distress range from the muscular system to the central nervous system.[40] Muscle system involvement is extremely common, with one of the most prevalent forms being headache.

In viewing the causes, responses, and reactions of stress, it should be evident that this topic concerns virtually everyone. The previous material should assist you in attributing events to stressors. The following section will introduce possible courses of action for coping with stress.

Stress Management

Working can produce distress and eustress. In addition to the causative factors previously discussed, characteristics of conditions in which eustress and distress are present will be examined.

 Building Comprehension Exercise begins on following page

Analyzing Work-related Stress Reactions

How often have you experienced the following reactions that were caused by work-related distress?

	Frequently	Occasionally	Rarely	Never
Yelling at patients/clients or treating them rudely				
Yelling at or treating a manager rudely				
Yelling at coworkers or treating them rudely				
Substance abuse				
Missing work when you are not sick				
Being late for work or returning from breaks late				
Quitting a job				
Producing less work, slowing your pace				
Having decreased level of motivation for work				
Feeling indifferent toward your work				
Having increased numbers of accidents				
Gastrointestinal problems				
Increased blood pressure, or pulse rate, or both				
Headache				
Insomnia				

Analyze your responses. What conclusion can you draw from your results?

_____

_____

_____

End of exercise. Text continues on following page.

Finally, an introduction to stress management techniques will be provided.

RECOGNIZING EUSTRESS AND DISTRESS CONDITIONS

People may exhibit many of the symptoms already identified as reactions to distress even when they are not confronted with *work* stress. The reactions may be due to stress not associated with work stress, or the reactions may not be stress related at all. Most of the signs of distress reactions have been introduced. Table 12–1 summarizes them. However, many of the signs of eustress from work have not been presented. They are summarized in Table 12–2. These two tables may assist you in arriving at a preliminary conclusion as to whether or not stress reactions are being caused by work.

If you are exhibiting signs of distress reactions, and yet many of the eustress examples of Table 12–2 are applicable to you, your reactions may not be due to work stress. If you believe that you are having distress reactions from work, you should discuss your work situation with your boss or a representative from your employee assistance program. If your distress reactions do *not* seem to be caused by work, you should seek assistance on your own (you may still be able to receive help from an employee assistance program).

STRESS MANAGEMENT RECOMMENDATIONS

Stress management can range from minimizing or reducing distress in general to professionally supervised efforts to manage serious stress-related problems. The following discussion is meant only as a guide to what is possible. Any problems that go beyond a superficial level should be addressed by trained professionals.

The following are elements of the working environment that can be used to minimize distress.[41] They include:

TABLE 12–1 • DISTRESS SITUATION CHARACTERISTICS

Insomnia and other sleep disturbances

Asthma and other breathing problems

Skin rashes

Anorexia and other eating disturbances

Ulcers

Nausea

Irritable bowel syndrome (small-bowel and colon spasms)

Increased pulse rate and blood pressure

Headache, neck ache, and backache

Dry mouth or throat, or both

TABLE 12–2 • EUSTRESS SITUATION CHARACTERISTICS

The employee:

Performs job successfully.

Maintains positive attitude and outlook on life.

Actively listens to others.

Responds to others, and they respond in turn.

Easily and empathetically communicates with clients, coworkers, or managers.

Laughs, smiles, and jokes with others.

Applies knowledge and creative abilities.

Recognizes the contributions of others.

Maintains productivity; that is, high quantity and quality of work.

BUILDING COMPREHENSION EXERCISE 12–3

Performing Stress Analysis

Part 1

Chart your stress and create a stress management plan for yourself. Use this chart (make copies if necessary) to register your stress level over a number of days (14–28). Measure your stress every hour and write down what you were doing at the time. Check the HD column if you felt high levels of distress, MD for moderate levels of distress, N for neutral, ME for moderate levels of eustress, and HE for high levels of eustress. Analyze the results, looking for patterns (regularly occurring stress) or highly distressful situations. Develop a plan to reduce or gain relief from the distressful time or activity.

Date _____	Activity	HD	MD	N	ME	HE
5 AM						
6 AM						
7 AM						
8 AM						
9 AM						
10 AM						
11 AM						
12 noon						
1 PM						
2 PM						
3 PM						
4 PM						
5 PM						
6 PM						
7 PM						
8 PM						

Exercise continues on following page ❀ ❀ ❀

Date ____	Activity	HD	MD	N	ME	HE
9 PM						
10 PM						
11 PM						
12 midnight						
1 AM						
2 AM						
3 AM						
4 AM						

Part 2

Analyze your results and create a stress management plan. Separate distress-creating factors into work-related and non-work-related if necessary. Remember that this chapter is intended only as an introduction; seek additional or professional help if necessary.

End of exercise. Text continues on following page.

- Design of the work environment
- Work equipment
- Good sound, light, and ventilation conditions
- Established safety precautions
- Adequate safety equipment
- Risk-reduction programs
- Task variety
- Worker independence
- Opportunities for social contacts at work
- Opportunities for personal development

Many of these factors have been discussed in previous chapters (see, for example, Chap. 2).

There are also things that should be avoided to minimize work distress.[42] They include:

- Work pace that is controlled mechanically
- Rapid, repetitive work motions
- Inflexible work methods
- Controlled pace that also requires a high degree of concentration
- Tasks that use or require little knowledge, initiative, or responsibility
- Work situations with few interactions with people
- Dictatorial supervision
- High levels of noise or other hazards

There are also stress management techniques that can be used on and off the job. Both of these start at the same point, however, The first step is to identify stressors.[43] The second step is to identify the impact of the stressors. Find out which are causing distress and which cause the most distress. Third, resolve to do something about a detrimental situation. This means not accepting the status quo. It means deciding to make a *change*. And fourth, take action. Do not just say you will do something—actually go out and do it. This action includes the major step of getting training or professional help when needed.

Other stress reduction actions that can be taken at work include receiving skills training when needed.[44] Lack of support from managees or coworkers can be a cause of distress. If so, take the necessary action to correct any deficiencies or to improve needed skills. If you feel you are too busy to do this, you may need time management skills.[45] The pace of the work from poor planning or organization may be the cause of your distress. The final on-the-job technique to minimize stress involves this book, especially Chapter 10, Change.[46] Applying the material that has been presented here may

reduce stress by clarifying your role in the workplace and by explaining the functioning of the working environment in general.

There are also techniques that can be applied outside of work, the first of which is to know yourself.[47] It is important for you to identify not only those stressors that cause distress but also your limitations.

It is important to have activities outside of work. Many people look to work to answer *all* of their needs, but it is unlikely that any work situation can be completely fulfilling. You should instead cultivate outside interests and hobbies.[48] Work time should give way to some time for playing and for entertainment.[49] Also, exercise is not only beneficial for physical health, but can produce eustress and negate the effects of distress.[50,51] Adequate sleep (something many Americans lack) is also an important part of stress management.

If these measures are not sufficient, it might be helpful to try meditation and relaxation techniques, which are beyond the scope of this discussion.[52] An alternative related to meditation is biofeedback, although monitoring equipment and professional assistance is required.[53] And once again, professional intervention by trained psychiatrists, psychologists, or stress management experts may be necessary.[54]

Summary

This chapter has provided a rudimentary discussion of stress and stress management. It has concentrated on work-related stress, identified work stressors and environmental factors to seek and to avoid, and shown that there are methods for managing stress. The basic objective has been to show that stress and stress reactions are common, but it is possible to develop your own strategies or seek out assistance to cope with both.

REFERENCES

1. Selye, H: Stress Without Distress. Harper & Row, New York, 1974, p 8.
2. Ibid, p 14.
3. Ibid, p 20.
4. Ibid, p 18.
5. Selye, H: The Stress of Life. McGraw-Hill, New York, 1976, p 74.
6. Selye, Stress Without Distress, p 37.
7. Selye, The Stress of Life, p 408.
8. Selye, The Stress of Life, p 408.
9. Selye, The Stress of Life, p 450.
10. Selye, The Stress of Life, p 450.

11. Selye, Stress Without Distress, p 41.
12. Levi, L: Preventing Work Stress. Addison-Wesley, Reading, Mass., 1981, p 76.
13. Ibid, p 77.
14. Ibid, p 78.
15. Selye, Stress Without Distress, p 41.
16. Schmidt, SM, and Kipnis, D: The perils of persistence. Psychology Today, November 1987, pp 32–34.
17. Lowenberg, G, and Conrad, K: Current Perspectives in Industrial/Organizational Psychology. Allyn and Bacon, Needham Heights, Mass., 1998, p 390.
18. McLean, A: Work Stress. Addison-Wesley, Reading, Mass., 1979, p 81.
19. Levi, p 35.
20. Lowenberg, G, and Conrad, K, p 391.
21. McLean, p 82.
22. Nelson, D, and Quick, J: Organizational Behavior. West, St. Paul, 1994, p 204.
23. Ibid, p 210.
24. Lowenberg and Conrad, p 391.
25. Vecchio, R: Organizational Behavior, ed 3. Dryden, Fort Worth, 1995, p 505.
26. Lowenberg and Conrad, p 391.
27. McLean, p 81.
28. Lowenberg and Conrad, pp 387–88.
29. Wolf, S, and Finestone, A (eds): Occupational Stress. PSG Publishing, Littleton, Mass., 1986, p 55.
30. Levi, p 71.
31. Ibid, p 72.
32. Ibid, p 80.
33. Ibid, p 73.
34. Ibid, p 77.
35. Ibid, p 78.
36. Ibid, p 77.
37. Ibid, p 78.
38. Ibid, p 77.
39. Ibid, p 78.
40. Ibid, p 76.
41. Ibid, p 86.
42. Ibid, pp 86–96.
43. Daft, R: Management, ed 5. Dryden, Fort Worth, 2000, p 491.
44. Ibid, p 494.
45. Vecchio, pp 512–14.
46. McLean, p 101.
47. Selye, The Stress of Life, p 405.
48. Greenberg, HM: Coping with Job Stress. Prentice-Hall, Englewood Cliffs, NJ, 1980, p 70.
49. Nelson and Quick, p 219.
50. Vecchio, p 511.
51. Vecchio, p 511.
52. Nelson, and Quick, p 219.
53. McLean, p 117.
54. Nelson and Quick, p 221.

13 ∘ Becoming Employed

∘ *Chapter Outline*

Objectives

On completion of this chapter, the reader will be able to:

☐ Describe the function and purpose of a résumé.

☐ Describe the parts of a résumé.

☐ Describe chronological and functional résumés.

☐ Describe the purpose and construction of a cover letter.

☐ List and describe the job application process.

☐ Describe various methods of locating job prospects.

☐ List the advantages and disadvantages of the various methods of locating job prospects.

☐ Describe the interview process.

☐ List guidelines for conduct before, during, and after an employment interview.

Most people do not look forward to the experience of searching for a job. As the previous chapters have demonstrated, the factors affecting you in the working environment are numerous and operate on each other and you in extremely complex ways. Not only must you select the situation you want, but also the employer must want you. Even if you find the place you want and are qualified to work there, you may not get the job. The economy may work against you, or the timing may not be right. For instance, you may hear, "We just this morning hired three new people—if only you had come in then!" Sometimes, serendipity seems to deserve as much credit as hard work. Still, every year millions of people conclude successful job searches, so there is equal cause for optimism. The reality, though, is that *nothing* you do will *guarantee* that you get the job you are after. However, there are things you can do that will increase your chances.

Preparing A Résumé and Cover Letter

You may not need a résumé to get the job you want, but it helps. A résumé performs four functions in fulfilling its single purpose. It serves as a record, an initial contact, an initial statement, and an inclusion-elimination device. Its single purpose is to ensure that you obtain an interview.[1]

Note that it is *not* the purpose of a résumé to get you a job. Some people think that if they mail out 50 résumés, someone will call them and offer them a job. That will not happen. Someone might offer to talk to you about a job based on your résumé, but you will not get a job through the mail and over the phone.

FUNCTIONS AND PURPOSE

The first function of a résumé is actually more for you than for prospective employers. A résumé is a *record*. It lists your education, work experience, and other items in an organized fashion. For someone with few work experiences, this may not seem like an important document. One can remember working for Wendy's one summer, Burger King the next, and McDonald's during the third. As more experiences are added, the dates, addresses, and so on can become more difficult to remember. A résumé is a place to keep this information so you don't have to remember it.

Résumés are useful as the *initial* contact between you and prospective employers. Along with a cover letter your résumé introduces you, notifies prospective employers that you are interested in seeking employment with them, and can save time. Sending résumés is faster than visiting a number of places, especially if you are looking to relocate out of state. And a résumé with a follow-up phone call can be an effective means of "getting your foot in the door."

A résumé is also an *initial statement*. It is often your very first impression. For this reason it needs to be perfect. A sloppy, misspelled résumé, hand-typed on an old typerighter (sic) that has a missi g "n" conveys a fairly strong message. It says, "I am not very precise, I am not going to take the time to do quality work, and basically I don't care much about work or my image." This is definitely not the way to achieve your goals.

The fourth function of a résumé leads directly to its purpose—it is an *inclusion-elimination device*. Employers look to résumés to form a list—a list of those to be included in the interview phase. At this stage employers are typically looking to narrow the field by eliminating those who are manifestly unqualified. Applicants may not be qualified because they are uncertified or unlicensed, lack the stated and needed experience, or are not available when the employer needs them (can't work nights or will not graduate in time). Final, or close, decisions are not usually made at this time. If your résumé presents a professional image and you meet the requirements, you will probably be contacted for an interview.

TYPES

There is no single best method for preparing a résumé.[2] However, speaking as someone who receives three to five résumés per week even when *not* looking to hire someone and who has had 525 people apply for one position, there is much to be said for the chronological résumé. This résumé type is discussed in this chapter as we examine some general rules for all types and some preliminary decisions to be made. The *preliminary decisions* consist of how many résumés to create, how the finished product should appear, and the type of résumé to use.

A decision on *how many* résumés to create does not refer to how many to have produced. It refers to varying the content of the résumé to better match the needs of a specific employer. There are two general methods for handling this. One is to have different résumés for different positions or employers. People with laser printers for their computers might select this option because custom-made résumés can be easily produced with high quality. The advantage to this method is the ability to create the custom résumé and to avoid being stuck with leftover, outdated résumés when your job situation or educational level changes. The disadvantage is the cost of a computer, laser printer, and good quality paper for those who do not have them.

The alternative is to have a general résumé coupled with custom-made cover letters. Specifics can be addressed in the cover letter, which is typed or printed for each employer, whereas the résumé can be professionally offset printed. The advantages are that the printer will assist you with format, and the résumé can be used for any position, making the modest cost of professional printing attractive. The disadvantage is the likelihood of being left with old résumés that are no longer usable.

Other preliminary decisions concern *how the finished product will appear*. These include decisions on print, paper, and white spaces. The best impression is made with a neat, professional appearance, which is most easily achieved with either professional offset *printing* from any of the numerous print shops listed in the telephone book or laser printing.

Decisions about *paper* are weight, texture, color, and size. Select a weight and texture to complement the printing method. A print shop will assist with selection; choose one of higher weight than regular typing paper (20-lb white bond is a good choice).[3] Select paper with the look and feel of quality. If you are using a laser printer, select paper texture and weight carefully. Some papers produce a sharper image than others; some curl during printing more than will others. If you are using an ink-jet printer, make sure the paper absorbs the ink properly and does not streak or blur. Paper color is another decision: white is the best choice. Off-white or light gray is permissible but not common.[4] The size of paper to use is letter size—8½ by 11 inches. Smaller sizes may be lost or discarded.[5] Some people have tried the longer, legal-size paper on the theory that when the résumés are held and tapped on the desk to even the bottoms up, the longer size will put the applicant's name above everyone else's, thereby getting it noticed. However, file folders are usually letter size, and when the longer paper doesn't fit, some managers just throw it away. It's best to keep gimmicks out of your résumé and let your education and experience speak for themselves.

The factor that actually contributes the most to the overall appearance of printed copy is not what's printed; it is the *white space* between and around what's printed. If you are using offset print, the print shop can assist you with this. If you are using a computer, you should experiment with different arrangements, margins, and spacing to achieve a professional, eye-appealing look. You may wish to test samples on people and solicit their reactions to different formatting. During this process, you should keep in mind the overall length of the résumé, which is discussed in the next section.

There are four *general rules* for creating résumés. These rules address length, spelling, content, and accuracy, and they apply to all types of résumés.

Résumé is French for "short" or "summarize." It is a *brief* description of educational and work experience. The length should be one to four pages: one is ideal.[6] This length is especially true for people new to the work world.

Spelling must be perfect. A résumé is a document that you should have spent time on, something you labored over. Misspelled words destroy this image. An employer might question the other abilities of someone who is unable to produce one or two perfect pages. If you have any doubt, consult a dictionary. If you are writing with a computer and word processing software, use the spell-checking and grammar-checking features. For additional grammar, usage, and punctuation help, consult *The Elements of Style* by William Strunk and E. B. White or *The Dictionary of Problem Words and Expressions* by Harry Shaw.

The general rule for résumé *content* is that you include your education and work history. However you do this, also include other materials to present yourself in the best possible manner. For example, a person who held two jobs while in his educational program—one flipping burgers and the other pumping gas—might consider this experience unimportant when applying for a position in health care. True, skills learned on these jobs might have little to do with medical diagnostics and therapy, but they do show positive assets. First, this person has work experience. Second, the experience includes working with the public. Third and fourth, he or she is motivated enough to work two jobs while going to school and has the time-management skills and discipline to juggle two jobs and an education. Although they may seem unrelated, these experiences show something about this person's character, a trait many employers look for.[7] The following are other points that employers look for that you should demonstrate in your résumé:

- A desire to work
- A work ethic
- Flexibility (in working times)
- Ambition
- Dedication[8]

Some ways in which you might demonstrate these qualities are listed in Table 13–1. These same points can be made in an interview, but it is best to document them in your résumé and then expand on them during the interview.

The content of the résumé should present the best possible picture of you to an employer, but it must also be *accurate*. Two major temptations toward inaccuracy are embellishment and omission.

TABLE 13–1 • EXPRESSING CHARACTER TRAITS IN A RÉSUMÉ

A desire to work	Holding a job(s) while in school
A work ethic	Previous work experience; holding more than one job at a time; holding a job(s) while in school; work-related awards
Flexibility (in working times)	Having worked various shifts and weekends; having attended evening or weekend classes while working days
Ambition	Previous work experience; promotions; advancement in professional organizations; advancement in community or volunteer organizations
Dedication	Long-term employment; membership in national or state professional organizations

Embellishment refers to inflating past positions or accomplishments. Don't. This practice in not only beneath the ethical standards of a health professional, but is too easy for prospective employers to verify in this information age. Don't say that you were the supervisor of the night shift at a convenience store, because when employers find out that the only person you supervised was yourself, the damage will be irreparable.

Omitting information is a little different. Because a résumé needs to be concise, you may have to omit the oldest or most unrelated of your experiences. You may need to omit very short-term jobs—ones that, for various reasons, may have lasted only a few days or a couple of weeks.[9] What should not be omitted are jobs from which you were fired or which you left on bad terms. Any gaps in your timeline will probably need to be explained. The best way to handle this kind of experience is to be honest if the question arises. Just because you were fired or left a job under less-than-ideal terms does not mean you were wrong. Employers make mistakes too. Include these situations, explain them, and show how you have learned from the experience and have grown since then.

There are two basic *types* of résumés from which to pick—the chronological and the functional.[10] The chronological lists experiences in reverse order, the most recent first. This résumé is the most common arrangement, especially so for new workers.[11] The functional résumé lists the skills you possess. It is not as applicable for the health professions because of the standardization of those professional qualifications, mainly through licensure and certification. However, a functional résumé may be useful when applying for a managerial position, an educational position, a cross-functional position, or a new profession that is still evolving.

As mentioned before, chronological résumés have at least one important advantage over functional résumés. Many people want to see your employment history in order. Functional résumés don't show this well. A problem can arise when someone is faced with reviewing many résumés. Obviously, the ultimate point is to sort through all the applicants and eventually emerge with the one that will be hired. So initially, the task is to eliminate people. When faced with 100 or more résumés, reviewers may be looking for any reason to reduce the numbers to something manageable. Having a difficult time sorting through a functional résumé and trying to determine if someone was continuously employed or how they advanced through different positions, may become a good enough reason to reject that résumé. I recommend a chronological résumé; however, if you really feel that a functional résumé would help you, include

a list of your employers, the positions, and the dates you worked, one per line, in reverse chronological order.

A *chronological résumé* is divided into sections. A fairly typical one would include:

- Identification
- Career objective
- Work experience
- Education
- Activities
- Honors

The *identification section* includes your name and address. However, if you will be relocating soon, it may be better to place your address on the cover letter. It is not common to include a picture with your résumé.[12] It is illegal for an employer to require a picture prior to your being hired. You may include one if you wish, but some states bar employers from having them in their applicant files.

A *career objective* is of greater importance for someone who is new to a profession because of the lack of work experience in that profession. If you are looking for the standard entry-level position in your profession, you can include your career objective in your résumé. However, there are some advantages to instead including it in the cover letter. The main advantage is that you can create a custom career objective for each employer or position. For example, your career objective could be slightly different when applying at a large- or small-size employer, hospital, clinic, or private office. Placing the career objective in the cover letter allows you to target each one.

No matter where it is placed, your career objective should show that you have given serious consideration to your professional career and the direction you would like to take. It should show a desire for growth. This "growth" is sometimes referred to as "advancement," but it does not necessarily mean a promotion to a management job. Growth (or advancement) means professional growth—learning. The career goal should show that you want to expand your professional knowledge and experiences. It should also show dedication to the profession. Ideally, everything in the career objective should be supported by the information in the résumé.

The section for *work experience* includes all full-time jobs and positive or relevant part-time jobs. The minimum information for each entry is the name and address of the employer, job title, and dates of employment. You may decide to outline your duties if they were significantly different from those that others with the same title had. The same applies to special responsibilities. The employer's phone number and your immediate supervisor's name can be included but are not required. The decision to include or exclude your salary level is a little more difficult. It is not common practice to give salary information; however, if it shows advancement or that your value to the company was increasing, you may wish to include it.[13] On the other hand, your reasons for leaving an employer are best excluded. If the question is of any importance, it can be asked in the interview. This will give you an opportunity to explain any difficult separations.

Your résumé should include a segment in the *education section* for each degree earned. This section includes name and address of the institution, dates of attendance, degree earned (or degree anticipated if you are currently working toward the degree and are close to completion), date the degree was earned (if not the same as the last date of attendance), major, minor (if applicable), and honors earned. Grades and grade point averages are not typically included. Special course work or extracurricular activities might be included if they are relevant to the position you are seeking. High school is not listed unless it is the highest level of schooling completed.

You may include schools at which you have concluded a significant body of work but have not earned a degree. Definitely include them rather than leave a large gap in your timeline. Rather than "degree earned," you might list "degree sought" or say nothing and simply list your major.

You may also include licenses or professional certifications you have earned under the education section or under a following section labeled "credentials."

The *activities section* can include professional, civic, or volunteer activities that demonstrate positive work habits, leadership, acceptance of responsibility, or the factors listed previously in Table 13–1. Relevance to the work world and the position you desire, plus brevity, should be considered here.

Honors may be handled in one of two ways. If all of your honors are academic, they are best included under the education section. This is especially true for those having attended only one school. If you have work or activity honors, you may include them in their respective sections or in this special section. People with numerous honors from different areas may wish to emphasize them within this special section. List the honor, awarding agency (if it is not obvious), and the year of the award.

Note that there is no section for personal information or for references. Most of what was listed under personal information in the past was either irrelevant or illegal for employers to ask about prior to hiring anyway. This includes height, weight, health, age, marital status, and number of children.[14] As far as references are concerned, few employers ask for them, and even fewer use them. If you feel compelled to say something about them, place one line at the bottom saying, "References available upon request."[15] The same applies to hobbies—do not include them. Some people feel that hobbies show that one is "well-rounded"; however, what you do on your own time is usually irrelevant to performing your job. Also, some people try to be clever when listing personal information or hobbies, which detracts from the professional appearance required of a résumé. Figures 13–1 and 13–2 are samples of chronological résumés.

Jane Doe

Work Experience:	General Medical Clinic, 100 N. State Street, Lemont, Illinois, 60439	
	Part-time Receptionist for three dentists.	August, 1999-present
	Full-time Receptionist for three dentists.	April, 1995-July, 1999
	United States Post Office, Red Desert, Wyoming	
	Full-time Mail Sorter and Mail Carrier.	June, 1994-January, 1995
	Home Depot, 75th Street and Woodward Avenue, Woodridge, Illinois, 60441	
	Part-time Cashier.	June, 1989-August, 1990
Education:	Elgin Community College, Elgin, Illinois, 60120. August, 1999-present	
	Associate of Applied Science. Major—Dental Assisting	
	University of Nevada, Las Vegas, 4505 Maryland Parkway, Las Vegas, Nevada, 89109	
	August, 1990-May, 1994	
	Bachelor of Science. Major—Anthropology	
Activities:	American Cancer Association, member 1996-present	
Honors:	President's List for four semesters. Elgin Community College	
	Outstanding Young Women of America, 1998	
	Who's Who in Anthropology, 1994	

FIGURE 13–1 • A chronological résumé.

John Doe

Work Experience:

McDonald's, Lincoln Highway, DeKalb, Illinos, 60115
Part-time French Fry Cook.   October, 1999-February, 2000
Full-time French Fry Cook.   March, 2000-June, 2001
Assistant Manager, Evenings.   June, 2001-present
Manager—Moe Howard

Larry's Spiffy Lube, 203 E. Roosevelt Road, Wheaton Illinois, 60187
Oil Recycler.   July, 1995-November, 1997
Lubricator.   November, 1997-July, 1999
Supervisor—Larry Fine

Education:

Northern Illinois University, DeKalb, Illinois, 60115.
August, 1999-May, 2002
Bachelor of Science in Physical Education, with Honors; Minor in Management

College of DuPage, 425 22nd Street, Glen Ellyn, Illinois, 60137
September, 1997-June, 1999
Associate of Science in Anatomy and Physiology

Wheaton College, Wheaton, Illinois, 60187
August, 1995-May, 1997
Doctor of Divinity

FIGURE 13–2 • Another chronological résumé.

The *functional résumé* is divided according to skills. Applicable educational and work experiences are listed under each skill. For example, the listing that follows could be an outline for a person applying for a position to direct a health-care educational program:

- Identification
- Teaching
  - Work experience
  - Education
  - Activities
  - Honors
- Professional
  - Work experience
  - Education
  - Activities
  - Honors
- Management
  - Work experience
  - Education
  - Activities
  - Honors
- Writing
  - Work experience
  - Education
  - Activities
  - Honors

Note that under the skills for teaching, managing, writing, and those specific to the particular health field, the categories are the same as in the chronological résumé.

COVER LETTER

A cover letter should accompany your résumé. A cover letter can have seven parts: the heading, salutation, introduction, body, closing, signature, and postscript and/or routing section.

The *heading* is the prospective employer's name and address and the date the letter is being sent. It is preferable to have a person's name rather than just "Director of . . ." or ". . . Department Manager." It is also preferable to have the person's correct title. Often, this information can be found in the American Hospital Association book of member institutions, from a state hospital association's similar publication, or from sources in your professional society.

The *salutation* is the "Dear . . ." line. The name used in the salutation should be copied from the first line of the heading and should be written in a formal style—for example, "Dear Ms. Smith:" rather than "Dear Jane,". Notice that after the person's name, the more formal colon is used rather than the informal comma. As with the heading, it is better to have a person's name here rather than "Dear Sir/Madam."

The purpose of the letter is set forth in the *introduction*. This first paragraph is relatively brief and

 Building Comprehension Exercise begins on following page

BUILDING COMPREHENSION EXERCISE 13–1

Creating a Chronological Résumé

Fill in the following information, and then create your résumé.

Identification: What name and address will you use?

_____

_____

Career Objective: Write three: one as if you were going to work in your health profession for your entire career; one as if you someday wanted to be a manager in your health profession; and a third as if you one day wanted to be an educator in your health profession.

Work in your profession.

_____

_____

_____

Work in your profession, and then become a manager.

_____

_____

_____

Work in your profession, and then become an educator.

_____

_____

_____

Exercise continues on following page ❧ ❧ ❧

Work Experience: List your previous employers, the positions you held, and the dates you were employed. Include the month and the year for each date. (For example, it's wrong to say you worked at a department store from 1998 to 1999 when really you worked the holiday rush for 4 weeks from December 8, 1998, to January 4, 1999.

Employer	Position	Start month/year	End month/year

Education: List your education after high school. List the school, dates of attendance (as with work experience, include the month and the year), and the degree. If you did not complete a degree, you may leave off this information or list it as "Degree Sought." Include professional certifications or licenses, too.

School	Start month/year	End month/year	Degree

Professional certification	Start month/year	End month/year

Activities: The only outside activities a prospective employer can legally ask you about concern professional organizations, so you may wish to limit this section to just that. If, however, there are volunteer or civic activities that reflect positively on you, consider including them if they are not too long. Do not include activities in social or religious organizations or hobbies because employers are not entitled to ask about these areas, and there is no need for you to introduce anything that could potentially bias an employer.

_____

_____

Exercise continues on following page ❧ ❧ ❧

Honors: You can include honors with the schools from which you received them if they are all academic. Honors draw more attention if they have their own heading, however.

_____

_____

_____

End of exercise. Text continues on following page.

should specify the position you are applying for and your immediate and future employment objectives.[16] You may also wish to describe how you heard about the job. The introductory paragraph should be about four sentences.

The *body* of the letter along with the employment and career objectives in the introduction are the areas that allow you to custom tailor your letter to the employer, position, or both. Possible topics include:

- Mention of your credentials that are particularly suited for this job
- How well suited you are for the position or for the organization
- Why you want to work for this employer
- Your key assets
- How you can help the employer or organization
- How your experiences prepared you for this position

At least one paragraph should refer to your résumé. You may wish to imply that there is more to you and your abilities than a brief summary like a résumé can demonstrate. In short, use the body to sell yourself to the employer.

The *closing paragraph* should demonstrate that you feel you have done an excellent selling job. It is used to ask for an interview, and it may even go so far as to suggest a time for the interview or to state a day and exact time when you will call for an interview appointment. The paragraph should contain four or fewer sentences.

The *signature section* includes a valedictory, your name in writing, and your typed name and address. The valedictory is typically "Sincerely," and is typed on its own line. Spaces are then left for your signature, followed by your typed name and address.

The last part is the *postscript and/or routing section*. It is an optional section that could include a postscript (P.S.) if you wish to give some information added for emphasis. In this respect it is different from a P.S. in a personal letter, where it is usually information that one forgot to mention in the body of the letter. In a cover letter it is used to draw attention. It should be something that is planned and calculated, not an afterthought.

The routing portion of the final section may include a line for enclosures and copies. An *enclosure* refers to documents that are sent with the cover letter. Typically the only enclosure is a résumé, which is not commonly noted as an "enclosure" on a cover letter. If it is noted, it appears on a separate line after the postscript or after the signature

section if there is no postscript. The abbreviation for enclosure is permissible: Encl. Résumé.

If copies of your cover letter and résumé are being sent to other areas within one institution, you may indicate this as the last line on the letter. For example, if the letter is being sent to a department manager with a copy to the human resources department, you may indicate this with "cc: Human Resources." The "cc" stands for "carbon copy," a term that dates back to the time before photocopies were commonplace. Figure 13–3 is a guide for a cover letter.

Methods of Job Searching

Once your résumé and cover letter are prepared, you must find places to send them or bring them to. There are six methods for locating leads on jobs. They are advertisements, the Internet, cold calls, word of mouth, networking, and employment or job placement organizations.

ADVERTISEMENTS

One of the first places people look for jobs is in the want ads. Sources include local and regional newspapers (especially the Sunday papers), professional journals, and professional periodicals. There are two types of advertisements that employers place. Open ads mention the name of the employer in the ad. Obviously, these ads provide you with valuable information so you may know the reputation of the employer (or be able to find out) and you will be able to contact them by letter and by phone if you choose. Blind ads do not mention the employer's name. You respond to the ad by mail through a post office box. There is nothing inherently wrong with blind ads, except that you must wait to be contacted and learn about the employer after sending in your résumé, rather than knowing some things beforehand.

THE INTERNET

There are numerous Internet sites dedicated to job listings like Jobs.com and Monster.com. Some offer assistance with résumé writing whereas others help you write an electronic resume that can be instantly e-mailed to prospective employers. Although the Internet is not yet positioned to replace other methods of searching for a job, it is certainly an important addition.

Heading

Name

Title

Department

Organization

Street Address

City, State, Zip Code   Today's Date

Salutation

Dear Mr./Ms. _____:

Introduction

I am writing in regard to a position in your department that was advertised in the

_____. This position (describe) is the type that fits well with my current goal

of (state 1 or 2). The reputation of your institution/office is one of _____ and

this coincides with y career goal of maintaining long-term employment with an orga-

nization that offers opportunities for professional and personal growth.

Body

(mention of your credentials and how well suited you are for the position; why you

want to work for this employer; your main assets and how you can help the employer

or organization and how your experiences prepared you for this)

FIGURE 13–3 • Sample cover letter.

COLD CALLING

Cold calling is the practice of visiting a prospective employer without an appointment. You have no idea whether they have a position open or not or whether a manager will be able to speak with you or not. Some managers will never see people this way. You may be able to leave your résumé or fill out an application in the hope that the manager will consult this file when a position does become available. Some will; some will not. Your only problem is that you never know which is which.

Cold calling can work, but a person using it is really relying on chance. Other options along this line include phoning first (saving you a great deal of time and travel), and mailing résumés for which you have no leads. Again, you may get lucky, but be prepared for a large dose of disappointment. Employing this tactic may well depend on your current position. If you are employed in the field, there are probably more efficient means of locating new employment. However, if you are unemployed, cold calling can't hurt, and if you persevere, you may be successful.

Closing

I have included my resume for your convernience. Also, in order to discuss this

situation and my qualifications in depth I will call you non (day and date) at

(time). in look forward to meeting you.

Signature

                                        Sincerely,

                                        Your Name

                                        Address

                                        City, State, Zip Code

                                        Phone Number

Post Script/Routing

P.S.   – (if any)

Encl. – Resume

cc   – Human Resources

FIGURE 13–3 • Continued.

WORD OF MOUTH

The main method of locating employment is through word of mouth. Seventy-five percent of all jobs are obtained this way.[17] Sometimes someone tells you he or she is leaving or planning to leave. Other times you hear from someone who has a friend who knows someone who just left a job. Whatever the scenario, word of mouth is essentially being in the right place at the right time to hear of a possibility. However, there is a more active method that can increase your chances of success.

NETWORKING

In essence, networking is active word-of-mouth job seeking. Networking involves developing personal contacts that can assist you in a job search and in your career in general.[18] Networks typically begin with the people you know—friends, relatives, and colleagues. They need not be in the same profession as you, nor even in the health professions. They may learn of job possibilities as

they seek health care, or they may read a local newspaper that you do not. However, this is only the beginning of the network. People successful at networking begin developing contacts early.

Network development beyond immediate family and friends can include:

- People in your professional organization
- Teachers
- Managers
- Sales representatives
- Community organizations
- Clubs

An excellent place to begin networking is through your local, state, and national professional organizations. Virtually every health profession has one. The greatest success will come from joining early and participating. Select events to participate in that will bring you into contact with new people.

Other contacts can be developed during your educational program and afterward. Take time to talk to and get to know teachers and managers. Often they are the first to hear about openings at other places because of their networks. It can also

 Building Comprehension Exercise begins on following page

BUILDING COMPREHENSION EXERCISE 13–2

Writing Cover Letters

Write three different cover letters for entry-level positions in your chosen health-care profession. Write the first one as if you are sending it to a 1000-bed university hospital that is noted for its research and medical education. Write the second to a 250-bed suburban hospital. Write the third to a small clinic in a rural county. First, write down how your three cover letters should be different; then write the actual letters.

Heading

_____

_____

Salutation

_____

Introduction

_____

_____

_____

_____

Body

_____

_____

_____

_____

_____

Exercise continues on following page ❖ ❖ ❖

Closing

_____

_____

_____

_____

_____

Signature

_____

_____

Postscript

_____

_____

Routing section

_____

_____

End of exercise. Text continues on following page.

be beneficial to become acquainted with health-care supplies and equipment sales representatives and equipment service and repair people. They travel widely and frequently hear of opportunities.

Contacts outside of the professional arena can also provide opportunities. Community organizations like volunteer groups and religious organizations have members throughout the job world. Also, members of clubs that you may belong to can also be of help.

The real power of networking does not come from people you personally contacted helping you. The real power of a network is that all of the people that you have contact with also have contacts of their own. And those people have other contacts. In other words, there is a geometric increase in the size of a network. For example, you are at parent-teacher night at your child's school and you mention to another parent that you will be graduating soon and looking for employment. That parent's sister-in-law sells medical supplies in another part of the state. Word reaches her to note any openings in your field. She does, word gets back to you, and you have a lead before the position is even vacant. This scenario may sound convoluted, but less likely chains of events have led to jobs for people.

Another factor in networking is that it is not necessary to impose on the people within your network if the contacts you have made are sound. You are not asking them to find you a job. You simply mention that you are looking and ask that if they hear of anything, to please let you know. You must carry the ball from there. Your contacts are not there to set up interviews for you or to even put in a good word for you. All you are asking is that they pass along any information they may come across to you. Most people are willing to help. Besides, you are also part of their network, and they may ask the same of you some day.

EMPLOYMENT AGENCIES

Employment agencies and job placement offices are a sixth source of job possibilities. There are two general types of employment agencies. One type charges a fee to employers, not to job seekers. The other charges you, the job seeker. Consideration could be given to using the first kind, the one in which you as a job hunter pay no money. However, this is probably not necessary for frontline positions in the health-care professions. The second kind, the agency that wants you to pay money, for whatever reason, should probably be avoided. Some of these agencies get their job listings by reading the local papers, cutting out the ads, and typing them up. With job trends in the health professions, and the predictions for increases in health-care employment, employment agencies can be considered a last resort.

Schools, states, and counties often operate job placement offices. Schools with active job placement offices are often extremely useful because they are free to the students from the school and often have excellent listings for entry-level positions. State and county run offices are also typically free to job seekers. Job placement offices often provide résumé writing and interview advice also.

Successful Interviewing

Virtually all employers interview job applicants, even though most interviews have little validity or reliability. Studies completed with people who agreed on the qualities needed for a position and in the methods for selection, which included interviews, did no better than chance in picking successful workers—and their selections had nothing to do with later job performance.[19] Another study demonstrated that selection success actually *decreased* when an interview was included. The best results were obtained by selecting people based on their credentials and results from objective tests.[20] Discussions with department managers may provide insight into the drawbacks of interviews.

The problem with interviewing as a selection tool quite possibly involves the kinds of things managers look for in applicants. The following is from an article discussing what some health-care managers look for in a job applicant:

- Neat, clean appearance
- Shows desire and displays a work ethic
- Flexibility
- Personality
- Ambition
- Dedication
- The person with the best presentation[21]

Note how many of these impressions are subjective. Furthermore, how do you demonstrate these in a 15- to 20-minute interview?

PREPARATION

The first step toward demonstrating these qualities and your general job worthiness is to prepare for interviews. This can be dramatically important because so few people bother to do it. Preparation can be divided into three areas: professional, physical, and mental.

Professional preparation includes education, experience, and activities. Educational preparation includes learning and experiencing as much as possible during your program. Good grades are important, as long as learning goes with them. Cramming or other tactics that increase grades without long-term learning will eventually catch up with people. In the health professions it is inevitable that the day will come when the material from your education will be needed on the job. It may not occur immediately, but some day it will.

Professional activities that can be engaged in during your educational program include joining local, state, and national professional societies. Participating in the society and attending meetings and seminars can also help in creating your professional network.

Physical preparation involves your résumé, cover letter, follow-up correspondence, and physical appearance. The résumé and cover letter have been discussed, and follow-up correspondence will be discussed at the end of the interview section. Regarding physical appearance, the guidelines for job interview dress and appearance are much the same as those for health professionals on the job. Dress professionally. Clothing should be conservative. Health-care uniforms are not necessary for the job interview. A business-type suit is appropriate. Hairstyles, makeup, jewelry, and scents should be kept conservative—the same as you would in a patient contact situation. For some interviewers, a large part of the decision to hire you or not is made in the first few seconds and is based on physical appearance. This is not fair, but it is true. You have only one chance to make a first impression, so make it a good one.

Another area of physical preparation involves knowledge of nonverbal communications. Your appearance, résumé, and verbal responses can all be negated by nonverbal signals. Avoid signs that convey nervousness such as fidgeting, restlessness, smoking, chewing gum, and pacing. Send confident, consistent nonverbal cues right from the beginning. Use a firm handshake. Sit upright, both feet on the floor, with your back slightly forward of the chair's back. Give more attention and eye contact than you receive, but don't stare at the interviewer. Maintain your focus on the business at hand. Do not become distracted by what may be going on around you. Above all else, pay attention and look interested. One way to gain control over your nonverbal communications is to practice being interviewed. Some people have even sought out interviews for positions they did

not really want just to gain experience in being interviewed.

Mental preparation for being interviewed can also be helped by practice. Mental preparation can involve three areas. These include your personal information, answers to typical questions, and information about the prospective employer.

Mental preparation begins with a thorough knowledge of your résumé and cover letter. Some interviewers will ask you about information they already have on your résumé. People who have lied on their résumé may reveal this by having difficulty when giving the information verbally.

Maybe the area where applicants have the greatest difficulty, and the greatest chance for improvement, is with answering questions. An interviewer's job is to make the applicant talk. As an applicant, your job is to sell yourself—to convince that prospective employer to hire you. To accomplish this exchange of information, interviewers ask questions. Although you will never know exactly what questions will be asked, there are some that are fairly common. Preparing answers for these will improve your presentation and separate you in the mind of the interviewer from all the people who do not prepare. The unprepared candidates will stumble into obscurity, but you will be remembered.

Interviewers want you to tell them what you think is important. Rather than answering, "Oh, I don't know," tell them what you think they need to know to hire you. Expand on your résumé. Explain the positive aspects for the employer if you are hired. Show that you have put some thought into selecting a career and planning for your future in this career. Accomplish this by putting some planning, time, and effort into preparing answers to the questions in Exercise 13–3.

You should also note that there are certain questions that are illegal to ask prior to employment. Sometimes they are asked anyway, perhaps because the interviewer is not familiar with the applicable laws. Handling these questions can be difficult for the inteviewee. Some people feel that if they do not answer, they will not be hired. Others may answer the question, and, if they are hired, say nothing (who will file charges against someone who just hired him or her?). If they do not get the job, they still might not file charges because this is an involved process that takes a long time, and there is usually no proof other than the complainant's word.

There are, however, more tactful ways of handling illegal questions. For example, a female colleague of mine was asked how her children would be cared for if she were to get the job (at this point the interviewer did not even know if she *had* children). This personal information is not something an interviewer can ask about. However, she handled it very well. Rather than answer the question, or rather than say, "It is illegal to ask that," she said, "Oh, if you're concerned about my ability to work these hours, don't be. I can assure you I can be here Monday through Friday from 8:00 to 4:30." Here, the potential employer's only legitimate concern in this area had been answered without a confrontation. The solution then is to prepare tactful answers to the illegal or intrusive questions just as you do for the commonly asked questions. The following personal information cannot be questioned before a person in a health profession is hired:

- Age or date of birth. But an interviewer can ask if you are the minimum age required to perform the job.[23]
- Grade school and high school graduation dates (could be related to age).[24]
- Maiden name.[25]
- Arrests.[26]
- Whether you rent or own your home.[27]
- Convictions, unless directly related to performing the job.[28,29]
- Training not related to the job.[30]
- Birthplace (or request for a birth certificate).[31]
- Parent's birthplace.[32]
- National or ethnic origins.[33]
- Native languages you speak. You can be asked if you speak a foreign language, but not if a foreign language is your native language, because that could indicate your national origin.
- Church attendance, religious affiliation, or religious holidays observed.[34,35]
- Marital status.[36]
- Spouse's occupation.[37]
- Number of children or intention to have children.[38]
- Child-care requirements.[39]
- Sexual preference.[40]
- Social or political group memberships.[41]
- Height, weight, or physical abilities unless directly related to the job, which would pertain to many of the health professions.[42]
- Handicaps or disabilities unless directly related to the performance of the job. Recently enacted legislation stipulates that applicants cannot be disqualified because of their disabilities. Fur-

thermore, employers will have to make accommodations for applicants who have disabilities. However, the extent of the accommodations is affected by the size of the employer and the vagaries of the Americans with Disabilities Act, which went into effect in July 1992.[43,44]

In addition, employers *cannot* request a photograph or a lie detector test. They can request credit information to verify past employment, but they *cannot* use creditworthiness as a basis for hiring or rejecting applicants. Agility tests and competency tests can be requested if the test materials are job related. Drug tests can be requested if the applicant is given written notice of the test.[45]

Some information that is related to the preceding items can be asked for *after* you are hired. For insurance purposes you can be asked:

- If you can legally work in the United States
- Your age
- Spousal information
- Dependent information
- If you are a U.S. citizen
- Membership in professional organizations
- Religious holidays you can work or accommodations that can be made
- To voluntarily supply minority status information to satisfy affirmative action plans[46]

Again, these questions can be asked only *after* you have been hired. Furthermore, you *must* be asked to provide proof that you can legally work in the United States *after* you are hired. If questions do arise, call the nearest office of the Equal Employment Opportunity Commission for advice.

The final area for mental preparation concerns what is usually the last part of the interview. Near the end the interviewer will usually ask if you have any questions. The typical response is, "No." This is a lost opportunity. Here, you have the chance to show that you are very interested in this position and in this employer. Do so by having some questions to ask. Some questions could be verification of information that you already know—"This is a Level 2 Trauma Center, isn't it?" or "There are six other employees in the department, correct?" This shows that you took the time to find out about this employer. This isn't a shot in the dark—you *really are* interested in working here. What you ask about may not even matter so much as that you did ask. Most people will not. You did. You will have the better chance of being remembered.

Other points to ask about may include ownership of the facility, number of locations, possibilities for advancement within the department, future

 Building Comprehension Exercise begins on following page

BUILDING COMPREHENSION EXERCISE 13–3

Preparing For An Interview

You are going to interview for an entry-level position in your health-care profession. Prepare answers to these common questions.[22] (Notice that none of these questions can be answered with a yes or a no.)

Tell me about yourself.

_____

_____

_____

_____

What are your long-term goals? Where do you see yourself 5 or 10 years from now?

_____

_____

_____

_____

What are your strengths?

_____

_____

_____

What are your weaknesses?

_____

_____

_____

Why do you want to work here?

_____

_____

_____

_____

Exercise continues on following page ❖❖❖

What can you do for us now?

_____

_____

_____

_____

Do you have children and how will they be cared for while you are working?

_____

_____

How did you become interested in this profession?

_____

_____

_____

_____

What three things do you like most about your profession?

_____

_____

_____

What three things do you like least about your profession?

_____

_____

_____

_____

End of exercise. Text continues on following page.

plans, and every manager's favorite, future expansion and new facilities and equipment.

CONDUCT

In addition to the preparation steps already mentioned, the way you conduct yourself during an interview can increase your chances of being hired:

- Arrive early. Do whatever you have to do to accomplish this.
- Remember the interviewer's name. You will probably be nervous so make a point to commit it to memory.
- Do not sit until invited to.
- Be attentive and courteous.
- Be honest.

There are also things you should not do:

- Do not smoke.
- Do not chew gum.
- Do not watch the clock.
- Do not try to be funny, overaggressive, or aloof.
- Do not appear overly concerned about money. Usually the interviewer will mention it, but if the interview appears nearly over and there has been no mention of it, then you may ask.
- Do not take notes during the interview. However, it is a very good idea to make some afterward.

There are also some steps to take for your own benefit. If it is not presented during the interview, ask to see a job description and a performance evaluation. These items will tell you about the job, how you will be evaluated, and the level of sophistication of the employer. If they are not available, how will you know whether or not you are doing a good job? How will the employer know? Also, ask when the hiring decision date is or when you can expect to hear from them. Some employers are very good about notifying all applicants about the job. Others call only if you are hired. This practice leads to a dilemma. Do you call or not? Some managers deliberately wait to see who calls. They believe applicants who call are the people who are truly interested. Others will become annoyed if you call. A third group will not mind a phone call. The problem is that you may not know which group a person falls into. The best action is probably to ask for a decision date during the interview. If you hear nothing in a few days after that, go ahead and call.

In addition to deciding whether or not to call prospective employers, you need to decide whether or not to write a brief note thanking them for their time. This practice is becoming more popular today, causes virtually no harm, and helps to keep your name on the employer's mind.

Finally, because health-care workers today often have a choice of employers, keep a card or a record of each employer, the impressions you had immediately after your interview, and other vital information. Then list the general job factors that are most important to you. List advantages and disadvantages of each employer. Compare all the factors, and make the best decision possible, given the information you have.

Summary

Finding a job is a difficult task, and there is no guarantee of success. However, it is possible to increase your chances of success. The key is to prepare. Many, if not most, people will not. They will apply, stand before the interviewer as if waiting for judgment to be passed, and accept the results, whatever they are. Following the guidelines for preparation that were given in this chapter can move you out of the role of waiting to be hired. That is, being well prepared can move you out of the position of waiting for someone (an employer) to do something (hire) to you. You can take an active role in selecting a position that meets your needs. These guidelines can give you more control. Preparation cannot guarantee success, but it can greatly increase your chances. All you can do is gain from being prepared; there is virtually nothing for you to lose.

REFERENCES

1. Powell, CR: Career Planning Today. Kendall/Hunt, Dubuque, Iowa, 1981, p 129.
2. Ibid, p 131.
3. Ibid, p 133.
4. Ibid, p 133.
5. Ibid, p 133.
6. Ibid, p 133.
7. Greer, KA: Managers describe ideal job candidate. ADVANCE for Radiologic Science Professions, June 22, 1992, p 5.
8. Ibid.
9. Powell, p 146.
10. Cicarelli, J: Job-hunting tips for executives. Management Review, June 1991, pp 39–41.
11. Powell, p 133.
12. Powell, p 133.
13. Powell, p 147.
14. Whitlach, K: Honesty best policy for job applications. ADVANCE for Radiologic Science Professions, June 22, 1992, p 7.
15. Powell, p 149.
16. Powell, p 166.
17. Cicarelli, p 41.

18. Powell, p 203.
19. Smith, HC, and Wakely, JH: Psychology of Industrial Behavior. McGraw-Hill, New York, 1972, p 163.
20. Ibid, p 167.
21. Greer, p 5.
22. Powell, p 228.
23. Whitlach, p 7.
24. Joel, LG, III: Every Employee's Guide to the Law. Pantheon Books, New York, 1993, p 28.
25. Ibid, p 23.
26. Whitlach, p 7.
27. Joel, p 23.
28. Whitlach, p 7.
29. Joel, p 27.
30. Joel, p 28.
31. Whitlach, p 7.
32. Roberson, C: The Businessperson's Legal Advisor, ed 2. Liberty Hall Press/McGraw-Hill, New York, 1991, p 60.
33. Whitlach, p 8.
34. Roberson, p 60.
35. Joel, p 25.
36. Joel, p 24.
37. Roberson, p 60.
38. Roberson, p 60.
39. Whitlach, p 7.
40. Joel, p 26.
41. Joel, p 25.
42. Joel, p 28.
43. Whitlach, p 8.
44. Joel, p 26.
45. Joel, pp 23–29.
46. Joel, pp 23–29.

Index

An "f" following a page number indicates a figure. A "t" following a page number indicates a table. A "b" following a page number indicates a box.